Bodybuilding

Cookbook for Women

A Smart and Easy Guide to Making 120 Tasty, Useful and Healthy Recipes with Photos Plus A 30-Day Meal Plan. Now You Really Can Transform Yourself into A Stronger, Healthier Person and Finally Have a Better Life…

By

Lindsay Dyer

Introduction

For those who are interested in women's bodybuilding, diet is an important part of the equation. In order to achieve the desired results, bodybuilding requires good nutrition and carefully controlled macronutrient intake. Different body types require different approaches to diet and exercise, so it is important for female bodybuilders to tailor their diet plans based on their individual needs. Additionally, it is essential for bodybuilders to have an understanding of their caloric needs and to create a balanced macronutrient ratio from whole foods.

Bodybuilding Cookbook Women provides a comprehensive guide to bodybuilding for women, with 120 delicious and nutritious recipes geared towards helping women reach their bodybuilding goals. Plus, the book includes a 30-day meal plan to help you get started on the right track. This cookbook is designed to make bodybuilding as easy as possible and give you the tools and knowledge to transform into a stronger and healthier person. By following the recipes and learning all the fundamentals about bodybuilding in this book, you'll be able to get your desired results without sacrificing taste or your time.

Plus, these recipes won't leave you feeling deprived because healthy food can be both tasty and satisfying. Through bodybuilding, you can create a lifestyle that is both physically and mentally rewarding, but the foundation starts with having the proper diet and nutrition. This cookbook provides a clear path to success and will help you get to where you want to be!

So, invest in your health and life, and get started on your bodybuilding journey with this cookbook today. With proper nutrition, regular exercise, and proper supplementation (based on your individual needs), you will be primed to reach your bodybuilding goals in no time. Plus, the tips, tricks, and advice provided in the book will help you stay motivated and inspired to really excel in your new lifestyle. Don't hesitate any longer; it's time to start making powerful choices that will ensure success — now is a great opportunity to start transforming yourself into a stronger, healthier person.

Table of Content

Chapter 1. Understanding Women's Bodybuilding Diet Plan

Women bodybuilders understand that proper diet and nutrition are just as important as training and exercise when it comes to muscle growth and maintaining healthy body composition. Eating the right foods with quality sources of nutrients can make all the difference when it comes to reaching goals and improving overall health and well-being. Eating the right foods will ensure that she has the energy needed to lift weights and perform other intense tasks with success. Thus, nutrient-dense, balanced diets are a necessity for women looking to achieve optimum bodybuilding success. Eating too much or too little can have an unfavourable effect on their goals, reducing the results they achieve in favour of an unhealthy lifestyle.

After all, the food a woman consumes is the fuel she needs to complete her training and make her bodybuilding goals a reality. Additionally, the right meals can also contribute to her long-term health goals, such as reducing her risk of chronic illnesses and disease.

For women, the bodybuilding diet plan might have some slight variations when compared to the standard diet plan due to a few reasons:

1. Women have different nutrition needs when compared to men, as their metabolic rate tends to be slower. This means they need fewer calories and rely more heavily on a quality nutrition plan to meet their needs. As a woman's goal is usually to build muscle and definition, it's important to focus on high-quality macro and micronutrients to provide energy and keep her on track with her bodybuilding goals. Additionally, supplements can be used to support the body's needs for extra energy, vitamins, and minerals.

2. Women can build muscle and definition faster than men, meaning they need to be extra mindful of their calorie consumption and nutrition quality. Eating the right number of calories in the proper macros is essential for this goal; otherwise, a bodybuilder may risk not achieving her desired outcomes. Creating a balanced diet that combines the right macro and micronutrients, as well as foods for energy, will help ensure adequate nutrition for the body without over-eating. Eating smaller meals throughout the day is also beneficial for metabolism and digestion.

3. Women are more prone to health issues like osteoporosis and so often require more calcium and vitamin D in their diets. Eating a well-rounded diet with plenty of fruits, vegetables, nuts, and seeds can provide these essential nutrients and support strong bones and overall health. Additionally, avoiding processed foods and focusing on eating nutrient-dense meals can help the body maintain the essential energy it needs to get through workouts and any additional activities. Finally, women often have different dietary restrictions, such as allergies or veganism, that may need to be considered when planning a bodybuilding diet.

4. It is important for women bodybuilders to stay properly hydrated and consume plenty of fluids throughout their day. Drinking at least eight cups of water daily is a great way to ensure that the body is functioning at its best and keep muscles hydrated and nourished. Hydration also helps to
regulate body temperature during intense workouts and can prevent fatigue, which can be detrimental to success in bodybuilding. Additionally, adequate hydration can help reduce inflammation caused by intense exercises, making it a key factor for bodybuilders of all levels.

5. Finally, bodybuilding as a woman requires a lot of dedication and hard work to achieve desired goals and long-term health benefits. Regular conversations with a nutritionist and personal trainer can help ensure that goals are set, realized, and surpassed. Equally important is learning about recovery and rest; this includes getting quality sleep and listening to the body so that it can energetically handle the rigors of a bodybuilding lifestyle. Proper recovery can help women reach all the desired fitness outcomes they have set for themselves while reducing their risk of injuries.

Chapter 2. Women's Bodybuilding Diet Macronutrients

Women's bodybuilding is a unique discipline that requires a specific diet and careful analysis of macronutrient intake. For those serious about bodybuilding, having a deep understanding of macronutrients will help maximize their workout and nutrition goals. Macros for female bodybuilding must be tailored to each individual's lifestyle, age, fitness goals, and the number of calories taken each day. In this chapter, we'll discuss macros and provide an understanding of how to use them correctly. Protein, fat, and carbs are the three main macronutrients that play an important role in a bodybuilder's diet. Each macro has its own unique benefits as a source of energy, and everyone should be aware of how these macronutrients should be balanced in their diet in order to achieve their goals. Women who are trying to gain weight should stick to a recommended macro balance of approximately 30% protein, 30% fat, and 40% carbs. This combination of macros will provide them with the necessary energy to fuel their body without sacrificing their ability to gain weight with enough protein.

Carbohydrates

Carbs are a great source of quick energy and should be consumed both before and after a workout. They provide the body with the fuel it needs to gain muscle mass and can help women retain muscle too. It is important that women choose complex carbs such as whole grains, quinoa, oats, and sweet potatoes over simple carbs like white bread and sugary drinks. Eating complex carbohydrates helps to stabilize blood sugar, encourages the body to burn more fat, and supports the production of hormones related to muscle growth, such as insulin and testosterone. Lastly, carbohydrates should be spaced throughout the day, with a higher percentage first thing in the morning and post-workout.

Protein

Protein is one of the most important macronutrients for bodybuilding. It helps the body build muscle, aids with the proper functioning of enzymes and hormones, and promotes healthy skin and nails. Women should aim to eat 1.5-1.8 grams of protein per kilogram of body weight per day. Quality sources of protein with a high biologic value include meat, poultry, fish, dairy, eggs, and vegetable-based proteins like lentils, beans, and nuts. Eating a diet high in protein helps women to build lean muscle and also aids with post-workout recovery. Protein can also help women to stay fuller for longer. Protein should be consumed throughout the day rather than all at once.

Fat

Fat is an incredibly important part of the bodybuilder's diet, as it helps to regulate hormone production and keep the body healthy. Women should be sure to get enough healthy sources of fat in their diet. Sources such as avocado, salmon, olive oil, nuts, and seeds are essential for maintaining good health and properly fuelling the body for bodybuilding. While fat should not make up more than 30% of total caloric intake, it is important not to completely eliminate fat from the diet either. With the proper diet, health and bodybuilding goals can easily be achieved when fat intake is set at the right level. Furthermore, eating foods rich in essential omega-3 fatty acids can help reduce inflammation, curb appetite, and decrease the risk of certain diseases. With a balanced diet consisting of both macronutrients and micronutrients, women can expect to reach their bodybuilding goals in a safe and healthy manner. Eating enough of the right macronutrients is essential for reaching peak physical performance for bodybuilders, so be sure to keep track of your energy needs when planning your diet!

Women bodybuilders, like men, take advantage of the cycle of bulking and cutting to attain the desired body look. Bulking is the period of time when bodybuilders increase their caloric intake to build muscle at an accelerated rate. This is followed by a cutting period, in which caloric intake is lowered and aimed for body fat reduction to reveal the new muscles. Depending on the goal, any female bodybuilder must understand the fundamentals of both dieting strategies.

Bulking: When bulking, the main training goal is to rapidly build muscle mass. This involves eating more calories than the body burns each day, as the energy and calories consumed can be allocated towards muscle-building efforts. Women should increase their daily caloric intake by a minimum of 500 to as much as 1,000 calories per day, usually in the form of healthy carbohydrates, proteins, and fats. In addition, women should also ensure that their nutrient intake includes adequate amounts of vitamins and minerals, so dietary supplements should also be considered.

Cutting: The cutting diet requires a reduction in calorie intake as a means of losing body fat and revealing newly built muscle. During the cutting phase, women should aim for a 500-calorie deficit from their baseline calorie needs; this will put them in a negative energy balance and help their bodies to start burning fat for energy. Macronutrients should be limited to a moderate number of healthy carbs, proteins, and fats, with most of the extra energy being sourced from low-calorie vegetables. As with the bulking period, dietary supplements may be needed to ensure adequate nutrient intake is achieved.

The Maintenance Phase

During maintenance, calorie intake should remain within the body's energy requirements. This helps to keep the body's metabolic rate functioning normally and prevents the body from entering a starvation state. While gaining, muscle should not be an endgame while in maintenance, eating adequate protein every day is essential to preserve and develop muscle tissue. When creating maintenance diet plans, female bodybuilders should aim to balance health and performance goals while their diet remains a source of fuel and nutrition rather than the centre of attention.

Ultimately, the bulking and cutting cycle should provide a basis for effective body sculpturing, allowing women to achieve their desired body shape and strength. Adjusting dietary intakes accordingly will ensure female bodybuilders get the most out of their efforts while still maintaining healthy lifestyles.

Ensuring an adequate combination of proteins, carbohydrates, healthy fats, vitamins, and minerals should be the main concern. This can guide Female Bodybuilders in meeting their goals and objective

Chapter 4. Why Make a Healthy Switch?

Women's bodybuilding nutrition is an important focus for those looking to build muscle mass, strength, and definition. When it comes to nutrition, making healthy changes is the key to maximizing muscle growth, improving health, and aiding fat loss. Women's bodybuilding diets should look beyond macro-nutrients (fat, protein, carbohydrates) and take into consideration vitamins, minerals, and a variety of other nutrients. So why should women make a conscious effort to switch to a healthy and balanced bodybuilding diet? Here's a list of benefits that will help you understand the importance of nutrition in women's bodybuilding:

1. **Disease prevention**: Beyond fitness, preventing illness is one of the main reasons people make healthy choices. Healthy diets are associated with a reduced risk of certain diseases such as diabetes, cancer, and heart disease. Eating a balanced diet full of vitamins, minerals, and other nutrients from foods like fruits, vegetables, nuts, and whole grains helps to prevent these illnesses. Additionally, adequate hydration helps the body to flush toxins and regulate body temperature.

2. **Better sleep:** The relative macronutrients consumed both during the day and before bed seems to play a role in sleep quality. Protein helps to travel from the stomach to the small intestine, where it is absorbed and utilized by the body. While carbohydrates and fat are utilized differently for fuel, the body seems to be more efficient in converting calories from protein into energy, which helps promote better sleep. Additionally, working to control diet-related inflammation helps the body regulate cytokines and hormones like melatonin, leading to improved restful sleep.

3. **Fewer injuries:** Diet is often overlooked in the fitness setting, but it is a major factor when it comes to injury prevention. Eating the right balance of foods not only helps to improve strength but also helps to protect the body from everyday wear and tear. For example, adequate hydration helps keep joints lubricated, which reduces resistance and wear on the tendons and ligaments. Eating nutrient-rich foods also provides the body with essential vitamins and minerals that can help minimize the occurrence of illness and injuries.

4. Sustained energy: The amount of energy we feel throughout the day is tied to our food and water intake. Complex carbohydrates and protein, for instance, can help control blood sugar and allow a steady supply of energy to the brain. Likewise, not drinking enough water can greatly inhibit our ability to transport nutrients around the body, leading to lower energy.

Anyone who is looking to get fit and tone their body knows that diet is a major component of that. The diet for women bodybuilders has unique guidelines to help shape and sculpt the female figure. To make sure that fitness goals that are set are achieved, it is important to remember a few tips that can help the process along. By following the diet for women bodybuilders and incorporating some of these tips, obtaining the desired body shape should be easier than ever.

1. Use a macro-counting app: Macro counting is a great way to track the nutrients that are eaten throughout the day. By using an app, keeping track of what is being consumed can come with ease. Plus, many apps have bodybuilder-geared nutritional sheets to make the tracking process go more smoothly. Apps like MyFitnessPal or MyMacros+ use powerful software to calculate the macronutrients in food. If you want to ensure that you follow guidelines based on your training phase, enter your meals into one of these apps. You can also use these apps to plan your meals and see the numbers before you start eating so that you can adjust meals to fit your macros.

2. Stay Hydrated: While many people understand the importance of water, not everyone knows the value it has with a bodybuilding diet. Water helps to flush toxins from the body and is needed for physical processes in the body. Drinking water also helps to decrease hunger, which can be beneficial when following a strict diet. Staying hydrated is key to having the drive to continue with an exercise and the determination to stay on track with the diet.

3. Meal prep: The concept of meal prepping has been around for years, and it is especially beneficial for those who are on a bodybuilding diet. By cooking meals in advance and portioning them into containers, food is ready to go when it's time to eat. This also helps eliminate the temptation to reach for an unhealthy snack, as the food is already prepared and ready at all times. Meal prepping also assists in keeping track of macros and calories, as only what has been made can be consumed.

4. Schedule your exercise: The importance of exercise cannot be stressed enough in order to achieve optimum bodybuilding results. Formulating an exercise routine and sticking to it will bring greater success. Many bodybuilders prefer to work out certain parts on different days. It is important to be consistent and get enough rest between workouts, as this helps muscle recovery and development.

5. Record your food intake: This is one of the most important aspects of building muscle and burning fat, as the diet for women bodybuilders needs to be tailored to individual needs. Tracking meals enables a better idea of how the body reacts and adapts to the diet. If the results are not meeting expectations, adjustments can be made to either the amount or types of foods consumed. By engaging in this practice, women will be better equipped to handle the challenges of the bodybuilding diet.

6. Listen to your body: It is important to listen to what the body is telling you. If something is off, it is important to recognize it and make necessary changes. Working out and dieting can be difficult, and it is ok to take a few moments and evaluate how everything is going. Taking ample rest, eating when hungry, and listening to the body are important components of the diet for women bodybuilders.

7. Speak with your doctor: Consulting a medical professional before beginning a new diet or exercise program is important as there may be underlying conditions that need to be addressed. Depending on individual needs and for safety, pre-existing conditions should be taken into consideration. Additionally, a doctor will be able to create a specialized program based on an individual's current level of physical health and provide insight into the best approach necessary to achieve personal goal.

Chapter 6. Breakfast Recipes

1. Banana Chia Overnight Oats

Preparation time: 5 minutes + chilling time
Cooking time: 0 minutes
Servings: 4
Ingredients:

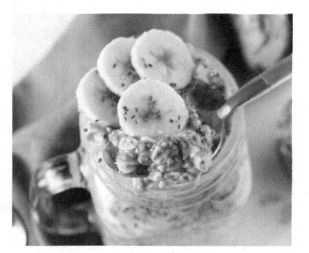

- 2 medium ripe bananas
- 2 ¼ cups skim milk
- 2 cups rolled oats
- 1 cup nonfat plain Greek yogurt
- ¼ cup chia seeds
- 1 scoop whey protein powder
- 1 tsp vanilla extract
- ¼ tsp ground cinnamon
- 2 tbsp almond butter

Directions:
1. In your small bowl, using a fork, mash the bananas well until smooth.
2. Mix in the milk, oats, yogurt, chia seeds, whey, vanilla, and cinnamon. Stir well, cover, and refrigerate within 4 hours or overnight.
3. To serve, top each portion with almond butter.

Nutrition: Calories: 432; Fat: 11g; Protein: 27g; Carbs: 58g

2. Sweet Potato and Turkey Hash

Preparation time: 10 minutes
Cooking time: 18-21 minutes
Servings: 4
Ingredients:

- 1-pound lean ground turkey
- Nonstick cooking spray
- 2 sweet potatoes, shredded
- ¼ tsp salt
- ¼ tsp freshly ground black pepper
- 8 large eggs
- ¼ cup chopped parsley

Directions:
1. In your large nonstick skillet over medium heat, cook the turkey for 5 minutes, breaking it up until cooked through. Set aside.
2. Coat the skillet with cooking spray and return to medium heat. Add the sweet potatoes and cook for 10 minutes, flipping gently, until browned and crispy.
3. Add the salt and pepper. Mix the turkey back into the skillet and gently stir. Transfer to serving plates or containers.
4. Coat the skillet with cooking spray and return to medium heat. Crack the eggs into the pan in batches and cook within 2 to 3 minutes until set.
5. Flip and cook for another 1 to 3 minutes until preferred doneness. Serve each portion of hash topped with eggs and garnished with parsley.

Nutrition: Calories: 454; Fat: 24g; Protein: 45g; Carbs: 15g

3. Protein-Packed French Toast

Preparation time: 10 minutes
Cooking time: 6 minutes
Servings: 4
Ingredients:

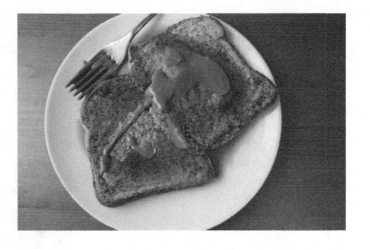

- · 2 large eggs
- · 8 large egg whites
- · ¼ cup unsweetened plain almond milk
- · 1 scoop whey protein powder
- · ¼ tsp ground cinnamon
- · Dash of ground nutmeg (optional)
- · Nonstick cooking spray
- · 12 whole-grain bread slices
- · ¼ cup ground flaxseed
- · ¼ cup peanut butter
- · ¼ cup maple syrup

Directions:

1. In your large bowl, whisk the eggs, egg whites, almond milk, whey, cinnamon, and nutmeg (if using).
2. Heat your large skillet over medium heat and coat it with cooking spray. Dip a piece of bread in the egg mixture, flipping to coat both sides.
3. Place the bread in your pan and cook within 2 to 3 minutes on each side, flipping once, until browned. Remove and set aside on a plate.
4. Repeat with the remaining bread, mixing the egg mixture well each time before you dip the bread to disperse the whey.
5. Thoroughly combine the flaxseed, peanut butter, and maple syrup in a small bowl. Top it with the maple–peanut butter spread, and serve.

Nutrition: Calories: 504; Fat: 18g; Protein: 33g; Carbs: 55g

4. Cottage Cheese Berry Bowl

Preparation time: 15 minutes
Cooking time: 0 minutes
Servings: 4
Ingredients:

- 4 cups of reduced-fat cottage cheese
- 6 cups raspberries, blueberries, or blackberries
- 4 tbsp slivered or chopped almonds or walnuts
- 6 tbsp unsweetened shredded coconut
- 6 tbsp maple syrup

Directions:

1. In your food processor, combine the cottage cheese and berries and pulse until mixed well.
2. Transfer to bowls to serve and top with the nuts, coconut, and a drizzling of maple syrup.

Nutrition: Calories: 888; Fat: 30g; Protein: 56g; Carbs: 72g

5. Baked Eggs with Smoked Salmon

Preparation time: 5 minutes
Cooking time: 15 minutes
Servings: 4
Ingredients:

- 2 oz smoked salmon, sliced thin
- 8 large eggs

- Sea salt & ground black pepper to taste
- 4 tbsp heavy (whipping) cream, heated and divided
- 4 tbsp thinly sliced fresh chives, divided
- Nonstick cooking spray

Directions:
1. Preheat the oven to 325°F. Spray the interiors of four 6-ounce ramekins with cooking spray. Line the ramekins with the smoked salmon.
2. Break your eggs one at a time into a small bowl, and pour them carefully into the ramekins on top of the salmon—season with salt and pepper.
3. Bake within 8 to 10 minutes until the eggs begin to set. Remove from the oven, and add 1 tbsp cream and 1 tbsp chives to each ramekin.
4. Return to the oven for a few more minutes until the edges are cooked.
5. Remove and let it cool. Once cool, remove from the ramekins. Serve.

Nutrition: Calories: 213; Fat: 16g; Protein: 16g; Carbs: 1g

6. Vanilla Blueberry Overnight Oats

Preparation time: 5 minutes + chilling time
Cooking time: 0 minutes
Servings: 1
Ingredients:

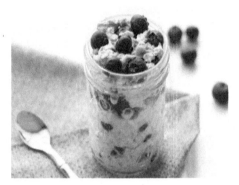

· ½ cup rolled oats
· 1½ tbsp chia seeds
· Pinch of salt
· 1 (1 oz) scoop of vanilla protein powder
· 1 cup unsweetened almond milk
· ¼ cup fresh or frozen blueberries

Directions:
1. Combine the oats, chia, and salt in a 2-cup glass container and stir well.
2. In a shaker cup, mix the protein powder and almond milk. Pour the liquid over the oat mixture and stir to ensure everything is well combined.
3. Top your oats with blueberries, put the lid on the container, and transfer it to the refrigerator overnight. Serve the following day for breakfast.

Nutrition: Calories: 466; Fat: 17g; Protein: 30g; Carbs: 49g

7. Spinach-Tomato Frittata

Preparation time: 10 minutes
Cooking time: 17-21 minutes
Servings: 3
Ingredients:

- 1 tbsp extra-virgin olive oil
- 3 cups sliced mushrooms
- 1 red bell pepper, finely chopped
- 1 garlic clove, minced
- 3 scallions, white & green parts, thinly sliced
- 2 tsp dried parsley
- Sea salt & black pepper to taste
- 2 large eggs
- 8 large egg whites
- 2 cups loosely packed baby spinach, chopped
- 1 cup cherry tomatoes, chopped
- ¼ cup crumbled feta cheese

- ¼ cup grated Parmesan cheese

Directions:
1. In a large oven-safe, sauté pan with oil over medium-high heat. Add the mushrooms and sauté for 5 minutes until tender.
2. Add the bell pepper, garlic, scallions, and parsley, then sauté for another 2 to 3 minutes, until the garlic is fragrant—season with salt and pepper.
3. Meanwhile, in a medium bowl, combine the eggs and egg whites and beat well.
4. Stir in the spinach and tomatoes, season with salt and pepper, then pour the egg mixture into the pan over the other vegetables.
5. As the eggs begin to set around the edge of the pan, allow the uncooked egg to flow underneath.
6. Cook within 8 to 10 minutes until the bottom is set and the top is almost done.
7. Meanwhile, preheat the broiler to high.
8. Sprinkle the cheeses over the eggs, transfer the pan to the oven, and broil for 2 to 3 minutes, until the cheese is melted.
9. Remove from the oven and let it cool. Slice into 6 equal wedges, and serve.

Nutrition: Calories: 290; Fat: 15g; Protein: 26g; Carbs: 11g

8. Banana-Nut Pancakes

Preparation time: 15 minutes
Cooking time: 4-6 minutes
Servings: 4
Ingredients:

- 1 cup gluten-free quick oats
- 4 large eggs
- 2 ripe bananas, mashed
- 2 tbsp full-fat coconut milk or other nut milk
- 1 tsp vanilla extract
- 2 tsp ground cinnamon
- 4 tbsp walnut pieces
- 4 tbsp raisins
- 2 tbsp coconut oil, divided

Directions:
1. Mix the oats, eggs, bananas, coconut milk, vanilla, and cinnamon in your large bowl. Stir in the walnuts and raisins.
2. In your large skillet over medium heat, heat ½ tablespoon of coconut oil.
3. Scoop ½ cup of batter into the pan and spread out with a fork, if needed.
4. Cook for 2 to 3 minutes until the edges of the pancake start to brown.
5. Flip and cook the other side for 2 to 3 minutes more until cooked through.
6. Repeat with the remaining batter. Let the pancakes cool on a baking sheet. Serve.

Nutrition: Calories: 355; Fat: 20g; Protein: 11g; Carbs: 37g

9. Egg, And Spinach Burrito

Preparation time: 10 minutes
Cooking time: 3-6 minutes
Servings: 2
Ingredients:

- Nonstick cooking spray
- 4 large eggs
- 4 large egg whites
- 1½ cups cooked brown rice
- 4 cups baby spinach
- 4 scallions, both white & green parts, chopped

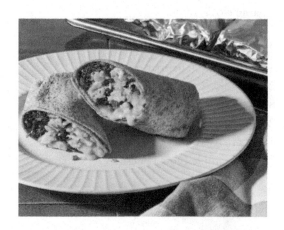

- 1 tbsp crumbled feta cheese
- 2 large whole-wheat tortillas
- ½ cup salsa

Directions:
1. Heat a medium skillet over medium-high heat and coat it with cooking spray.
2. In a small bowl, scramble the eggs and egg whites. Add them to the skillet and cook for 2 to 4 minutes, stirring, until mostly set.
3. Add the rice, spinach, and scallions and stir within 1 to 2 minutes until the spinach is wilted. Stir in the feta and mix to combine.
4. Divide the eggs between the tortillas, fold them on the sides, and roll them up to form a burrito. Cut in half and serve with salsa.

Nutrition: Calories: 602; Fat: 14g; Protein: 33g; Carbs: 80g

10. Ham And Feta Quiche

Preparation time: 10 minutes
Cooking time: 45 minutes
Servings: 4
Ingredients:

- Nonstick cooking spray
- 4 large eggs
- 1½ cups egg whites
- 1 cup reduced-fat cottage cheese (1%)
- 5 bacon slices, cooked & crumbled
- ½ cup finely chopped extra-lean ham
- ¼ cup crumbled feta cheese
- ½ onion, finely chopped
- 1 green bell pepper, finely chopped
- ½ tsp sea salt
- ¼ tsp freshly ground black pepper

Directions:
1. Preheat the oven to 350°F. Coat the bottom and sides of an 8-by-8-inch square glass baking dish with nonstick cooking spray.
2. In a large bowl, combine the eggs, egg whites, cottage cheese, bacon, ham, feta, onion, bell pepper, salt, and pepper.
3. Pour the mixture into your baking dish. Bake within 45 minutes or until the center is set.
4. Remove and let it cool. Cut into 8 equal pieces, and serve.

Nutrition: Calories: 322; Fat: 18g; Protein: 33g; Carbs: 6g

11. Vanilla Protein Crepes

Preparation time: 10 minutes
Cooking time: 3-4 minutes
Servings: 10 small crepes
Ingredients:

- 1½ cups unsweetened vanilla almond milk, + more if needed
- 1½ cups gluten-free rolled oats
- 1 scoop vanilla protein powder
- 1 large egg
- 3 tbsp egg whites
- 2 tsp coconut sugar
- 1 tsp vanilla extract

- ½ tsp ground cinnamon
- Pinch of sea salt

Directions:
1. In a blender, combine the milk, oats, protein powder, egg, egg whites, sugar, vanilla, cinnamon, and salt.
2. Blend until smooth. If needed, add more milk.
3. Heat your large nonstick skillet over medium-high heat.
4. Pour about ½ cup of the batter into the pan, tilting it in a circular motion to spread the crepe out as much as possible.
5. Cook for 2 minutes, until it bubbles, flip and cook for another minute or two on the other side. Repeat with the remaining crepe batter. Serve.

Nutrition: Calories: 312; Fat: 9g; Protein: 23g; Carbs: 36g

12. Egg and Canadian Bacon Cups

Preparation time: 5 minutes
Cooking time: 18-20 minutes
Servings: 6
Ingredients:

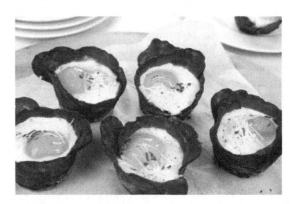

- 6 large eggs
- 12 slices nitrate-free Canadian bacon
- Pinch of salt & ground black pepper

Directions:
1. Preheat the oven to 350°F. Spray a large muffin tin with nonstick cooking spray.
2. Put 2 slices of Canadian bacon into each tin and shape them into cups.
3. Crack one egg into each cup and season with salt and black pepper.
4. Bake within 18 to 20 minutes or until the centres of the eggs are set and firm. Serve warm.

Nutrition: Calories: 264; Fat: 12g; Protein: 34g; Carbs: 3g

13. Breakfast Spinach Shakshuka

Preparation time: 10 minutes
Cooking time: 15-18 minutes
Servings: 4
Ingredients:

- 1 tbsp extra-virgin olive oil
- 1 small yellow onion, chopped
- 1 medium red bell pepper, seeded & chopped
- 3 garlic cloves, minced
- 2 (15-oz) cans of diced tomatoes
- 2 cups grated carrots
- 1½ tsp paprika
- 1 tsp ground cumin
- ½ tsp salt
- 4 cups chopped spinach
- 8 large eggs
- 8 large egg whites
- ½ cup chopped parsley

Directions:
1. In your large skillet, heat the oil over medium heat. Cook the onion and bell pepper for 5 minutes, occasionally stirring, until softened.

2. Add the garlic and sauté within 30 seconds, until fragrant.
3. Add the tomatoes and carrots and mix well. Stir in the paprika, cumin, and salt. Let it simmer and cook for 5 minutes until slightly thickened.
4. Stir in the spinach. Then, using a large spoon, make 8 wells in the mixture, evenly spaced throughout the skillet.
5. Crack an egg into each well and pour the egg whites on top of the eggs. Cover and cook for 5 to 8 minutes, until cooked to your desired doneness.
6. Garnish with chopped parsley and serve.

Nutrition: Calories: 327; Fat: 15g; Protein: 24g; Carbs: 24g

14. Apple-Oat Protein Muffins

Preparation time: 15 minutes + cooling time
Cooking time: 35 minutes
Servings: 12 muffins
Ingredients:

- 2½ cups rolled oats
- 3 tbsp coconut sugar
- 2 tbsp chia seeds
- 2½ scoops vanilla vegan protein powder
- 1 tbsp ground cinnamon
- Pinch of sea salt
- 2 cups unsweetened vanilla almond milk
- ½ cup unsweetened applesauce
- ½ cup egg whites
- 1 tbsp vanilla extract
- 2 tbsp coconut oil, melted
- 2 cups peeled and finely chopped apples

Directions:

1. Preheat the oven to 375°F. Line a 12-cup muffin tin with silicone baking cups.
2. Mix the oats, coconut sugar, chia seeds, protein powder, cinnamon, and salt in your large bowl.
3. Whisk together the almond milk, applesauce, egg whites, and vanilla in your medium bowl.
4. Pour the wet mixture into your dry mixture, then stir in the coconut oil and the apples. Divide the batter evenly among your muffin cups.
5. Bake within 35 minutes, or until a toothpick inserted comes out clean, and remove from the oven.
6. Remove the muffin cups from the pan and let them cool on a wire rack within 30 minutes. Serve.

Nutrition: Calories: 151; Fat: 6g; Protein: 7g; Carbs: 21g

15. Sausage-Egg Scramble

Preparation time: 5 minutes
Cooking time: 7-8 minutes
Servings: 2
Ingredients:

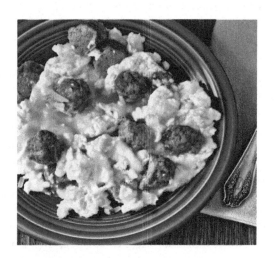

- 2 large eggs
- 4 large egg whites
- 2 tbsp reduced-fat cream (5%)
- Pinch ground cayenne pepper to taste
- Sea salt & ground black pepper
- ½ tbsp coconut oil or butter
- 2 pre-cooked turkey sausages, diced
- 2 tbsp finely chopped scallions, white and green parts
- ¼ cup grated cheddar cheese

Directions:
1. Mix the eggs, egg whites, cream, and cayenne in a medium bowl. Whisk until well blended, and season with salt and pepper. Set aside.
2. In your medium skillet over medium-high heat, melt the coconut oil. Add the sausages and cook for 3 to 4 minutes, until browned.
3. Add the scallions and sauté for 3 minutes until translucent.
4. Pour the egg mixture into your pan and cook for 1 minute, stirring frequently.
5. Just before the eggs are fully cooked, sprinkle on the cheese. Continue cooking until the cheese has melted. Serve.

Nutrition: Calories: 477; Fat: 36g; Protein: 35g; Carbs: 3g

16. Breakfast Greek Yogurt Parfait

Preparation time: 5 minutes
Cooking time: 0 minutes
Servings: 2
Ingredients:
- 2 cups nonfat plain Greek yogurt
- 2 tbsp creamy unsweetened peanut butter
- 1 tbsp honey
- 1 tsp vanilla extract
- 1 large banana, sliced
- ¼ cup granola

Directions:
1. Mix the yogurt, peanut butter, honey, and vanilla in a medium bowl. Stir until completely combined and smooth.
2. Into each of 2 airtight glass containers, place a heaping cup
3. of yogurt, topped with half a banana and 2 tbsp granola. Serve.

Nutrition: Calories: 343; Fat: 16g; Protein: 31g; Carbs: 47g

17. Eggs and Tomato Breakfast Melts

Preparation time: 10 minutes
Cooking time: 3-5 minutes
Servings: 1
Ingredients:
- 1 whole-grain English muffin, split
- ½ tsp extra-virgin olive oil
- 2 scallions, finely chopped & divided
- 4 egg whites, whisked
- Salt & ground black pepper, to taste
- ¼ cup halved cherry tomatoes
- ¼ cup shredded Mexican cheese blend

Directions:
1. Preheat the broiler.
2. Add the English muffin halves into a toaster and toast until golden brown. Place onto a baking sheet.
3. Warm the oil in a small nonstick skillet over medium heat. Add half the scallions and sauté for 2 to 3 minutes.
4. Add the egg whites, salt, and pepper to the pan. Stir with a spatula until eggs are fully cooked; remove from heat.
5. Layer the muffin halves with scrambled egg whites, tomatoes, and cheese. Broil for 1 to 2 minutes until the
6. cheese melts.
7. Transfer breakfast melts to a plate, garnish with remaining scallions, and serve.

Nutrition: Calories: 335; Fat: 12g; Protein: 27g; Carbs: 31g

18. Tempeh & Kale Breakfast Skillet

Preparation time: 5 minutes
Cooking time: 16-19 minutes
Servings: 3
Ingredients:

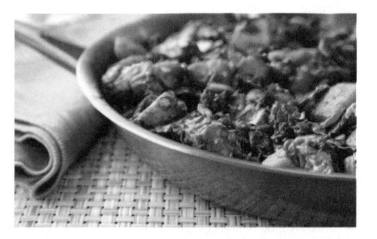

- 1 tbsp olive oil or coconut oil
- 1 white onion, chopped
- Pinch of salt
- 2 garlic cloves, minced
- Pinch of red chili flakes (optional)
- 1 (9-oz) package of tempeh, chopped
- 3 tbsp soy sauce
- 2 tbsp apple cider vinegar
- 4 cups chopped kale
- Freshly ground black pepper to taste

Directions:

1. In a medium skillet, warm the oil over medium-high heat. Add the onion and salt, then sauté for 5 minutes until the onions are translucent.
2. Add the garlic and chili flakes (if using) and cook for 1 minute more.
3. Add the tempeh, soy sauce, and vinegar, and give it a good stir. Cover and steam the tempeh for 8 to 10 minutes, stirring often.
4. Stir in the kale and cook uncovered for 2 to 3 minutes or until the kale has wilted. Season with salt and pepper, if desired. Serve.

Nutrition: Calories: 279; Fat: 14g; Protein: 19g; Carbs: 24g

19. Blueberry Cobbler Oatmeal

Preparation time: 5 minutes + soaking time
Cooking time: 5-6 minutes
Servings: 3
Ingredients:

- 1 cup rolled oats
- 1½ cups unsweetened vanilla cashew or almond milk
- Pinch of sea salt
- 1 cup water
- 1 to 1½ tbsp tahini
- 1½ tbsp pure maple syrup
- 1 tbsp ground flaxseed
- 1 tsp vanilla extract
- 1½ cups fresh blueberries, divided
- 3 tbsp almond butter, divided
- 1½ tbsp chopped pecans, divided
- 1½ tbsp chopped white chocolate, divided

Directions:

1. Combine the oats, cashew milk, salt, and water in a small saucepan. Let it sit for 5 minutes to soak.
2. Let it boil over high heat while stirring. Adjust to low heat.
3. Stir in the tahini, maple syrup, flaxseed, and vanilla, and continue to cook over low heat for another 5 to 6 minutes or until thick and creamy.
4. Divide the oatmeal evenly among 3 bowls. Top each with ½ cup of blueberries, 1 tbsp nut butter, ½ tbsp pecans, and ½ tbsp white chocolate, and serve.

Nutrition: Calories: 356; Fat: 19g; Protein: 9g; Carbs: 33g

20.Classic Tofu Scramble

Preparation time: 10 minutes

Cooking time: 25 minutes

Servings: 4-6

Ingredients:

- 1 tbsp olive oil or coconut oil
- 1 white onion, chopped
- Few pinches of salt
- 2 cloves of garlic, minced
- 1 tsp turmeric
- 1 (16-oz) package of organic firm tofu, crumbled
- ¼ cup nutritional yeast
- 1 tsp salt
- 4 cups spinach, tightly packed
- Freshly ground black pepper to taste

Directions:

1. In your large skillet, warm the oil over medium heat. Sauté the onions with salt and a splash of water, and cook for 5 minutes, often stirring until slightly translucent.
2. Add the garlic and cook within 1 minute more; then stir in the turmeric.
3. Mix in the crumbled tofu, nutritional yeast, and black salt. Cook for a few minutes, often stirring, to warm the tofu.
4. Add the spinach and cook until it is wilted—season with additional salt and pepper. Serve immediatly.

Nutrition: Calories: 191; Fat: 10g; Protein: 19g; Carbs: 14g

Chapter 7. Lunch Recipes

21. Grilled Greek Chicken Kabobs

Preparation time: 10 minutes

Cooking time: 6-8 minutes

Servings: 6

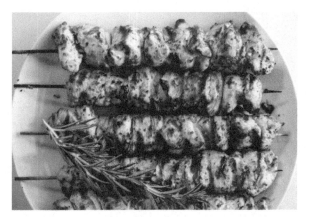

- Ingredients:
- 12- to 18-oz boneless, skinless chicken breast cut into half-inch cubes
- 6 to 8 fresh shiitake mushrooms, stem trimmed & cut into half-inch dice
- 12 fresh rosemary sprigs
- Sea salt & ground black pepper to taste
- ¼ cup extra-virgin olive oil

Directions:

1. Heat a grill to medium-high or preheat the oven to 425°F.
2. Skewer 3 pieces of chicken and 2 pieces of mushroom alternately onto each rosemary sprig. Season with salt and pepper, and brush with olive oil.
3. Grill the skewers over medium heat for 6 to 8 minutes or until any chicken juices run clear. Let it cool, and serve.

Nutrition: Calories: 293; Fat: 15g; Protein: 26g; Carbs: 12g

22. Veggie Fried Rice

Preparation time: 10 minutes

Cooking time: 34-41 minutes

Servings: 6

Ingredients:

- 2 cups basmati rice
- 1 tsp sea salt, + more for seasoning
- 2 tbsp + 1 tsp extra-virgin olive oil, divided
- 4 cups water, + 2 tbsp, divided
- ½ medium onion, finely chopped
- ½ red bell pepper, finely chopped
- ½ yellow bell pepper, finely chopped
- 1 celery stalk, finely chopped
- 2 small tomatoes, finely chopped
- Freshly ground black pepper to taste

Directions:

1. In a large stockpot, combine the rice, salt, 1 tsp olive oil, and 4 cups water. Let it boil.
2. Once boiling, adjust to low heat, cover, and continue to simmer within 25 to 30 minutes until the water is absorbed.
3. Meanwhile, heat your large skillet over medium heat. Add the remaining olive oil and onion, then sauté for 2 minutes.
4. Add the peppers, celery, and tomatoes and continue to sauté for 2 more minutes, stirring—season with salt and pepper.
5. Add 2 tablespoons of water, cover the saucepan with a lid,
6. and steam the vegetables for 5 to 7 more minutes, stirring occasionally. Remove from the heat and set aside.
7. Once the rice is ready, add the vegetables and stir to combine. Serve.

Nutrition: Calories: 270; Fat: 4g; Protein: 5g; Carbs: 53g

23.Baked Panko-Breaded Pork Chop

Preparation time: 10 minutes

Cooking time: 20 minutes

Servings: 4

Ingredients:

- 4 (4 oz) boneless pork chops
- ½ tsp paprika
- ½ tsp salt
- ¼ tsp freshly ground black pepper
- 2 large eggs, beaten
- 1 cup panko bread crumbs

Directions:

1. Preheat the oven to 400°F. Line a baking sheet with parchment paper.
2. Season the meat with paprika, salt, and pepper. In a small bowl, beat the eggs. Place the bread crumbs in your small bowl.
3. Dip the pork chops into the eggs, roll them in the bread crumbs, and place them on the prepared baking sheet.
4. Bake for 20 minutes, until the juices run clear and the breading is browned.

Nutrition: Calories: 241; Fat: 7g; Protein: 28g; Carbs: 16g

24.Lettuce Wraps with Smoked Tofu

Preparation time: 10 minutes

Cooking time: 35 minutes

Servings: 4

Ingredients:

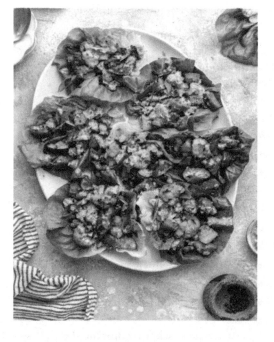

- 1 (13-oz) package of organic, extra-firm smoked tofu, drained & cubed
- 1 tbsp coconut oil
- ½ cup yellow onion, finely chopped
- 3 celery stalks, finely chopped
- 1 red bell pepper, chopped
- Pinch salt
- 1 cup cremini mushrooms, finely chopped
- 1 garlic clove, minced
- ½ tsp ginger, minced
- 3 tbsp soy sauce
- ½ tsp red pepper flakes
- Freshly ground black pepper to taste
- 8 to 10 large romaine leaves, washed and patted dry

Directions:

1. Preheat the oven to 350°F. Line your baking sheet using parchment paper or a silicone liner, then place the tofu cubes in one layer.
2. Bake the tofu cubes for 25 minutes, flipping them after 10 to 15 minutes. Set aside.
3. Meanwhile, warm the coconut oil in a nonstick sauté pan over medium-high heat.
4. Add the onion, celery, bell pepper, and salt, and cook within 5 minutes or until the onions are slightly translucent.
5. Add the mushrooms, garlic, and ginger, then sauté for 5 minutes until the mushrooms release water.
6. Adjust to medium heat and add the soy sauce and the red
7. pepper flakes.
8. Add the baked tofu cubes to the pan and sprinkle with pepper. Sauté for a few minutes more, until the tofu is coated with sauce and the veggies are tender.
9. To serve, scoop as much veggie and tofu mixture into each romaine leaf as you'd like.

Nutrition: Calories: 160; Fat: 8g; Protein: 14g; Carbs: 6g

25. Loaded Sweet Potatoes

Preparation time: 10 minutes

Cooking time: 5-10 minutes

Servings: 4

Ingredients:

- 5 (4 oz) sweet potatoes
- ½ cup nonfat or low-fat plain Greek yogurt
- 2 tbsp lime juice
- ½ tsp chili powder
- ¼ tsp salt
- 1 (15-oz) can of black beans, drained and rinsed
- ½ cup cotija cheese
- 1 cup fresh parsley, chopped

Directions:

1. Using a fork, poke the sweet potatoes a couple of times each. Place them on a plate and microwave for 5 to 10 minutes until tender.
2. Split four of the potatoes lengthwise, leaving about ¼ inch of flesh connected on the bottom. Dice the remaining potato into cubes and set aside.
3. Whisk together the yogurt, lime juice, chili powder, and salt in your small bowl.
4. Top the potato halves with the black beans, cheese, cubed potatoes, and parsley, and serve with 2 tbsp seasoned yogurt on top.

Nutrition: Calories: 348; Fat: 6g; Protein: 15g; Carbs: 50g

26. Salmon Salad Wrap

Preparation time: 10 minutes

Cooking time: 0 minutes

Servings: 2

Ingredients:

- 1 (5-oz) can of boneless, skinless salmon, drained
- ½ cup nonfat plain Greek yogurt
- ½ cucumber, peeled & chopped
- ¼ cup chopped red onion
- 1 garlic clove, minced
- ½ tsp dill weed
- 2 large whole-wheat tortillas
- 2 cups baby spinach

Directions:

1. Mix the salmon, yogurt, cucumber, onion, garlic, and dill in a large bowl.
2. Divide the mixture between the tortillas and add 1 cup of spinach to each. Fold the sides in and roll up the tortillas.

Nutrition: Calories: 319; Fat: 8g; Protein: 28g; Carbs: 38g

27. Vegetable and Beef Skewers

Preparation time: 15 minutes

Cooking time: 6-10 minutes

Servings: 4

Ingredients:

- 1 pound flank steak, cut into 2-inch pieces
- 3 tbsp lemon juice
- ½ tsp dried thyme

- ½ tsp dried oregano
- ¾ tsp salt
- ½ tsp freshly ground black pepper
- 1 red bell pepper, seeded & cut into 2-inch squares
- 1 green bell pepper, seeded & cut into 2-inch squares
- ¾ pound white button mushrooms, stems removed
- Nonstick cooking spray
- 4 cups cooked brown rice

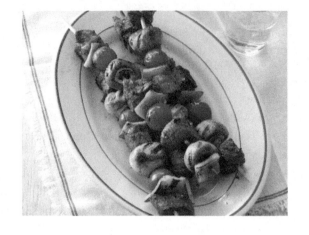

Directions:
1. In a large bowl, combine the flank steak, lemon juice, thyme, oregano, salt, and pepper. Stir in the bell peppers, mushrooms, and onion.
2. Thread the meat and vegetables onto skewers, alternating them.
3. Heat your grill pan over medium-high heat and coat lightly with cooking spray.
4. Add the skewers to the pan and cook on each side within 3 to 5 minutes, flipping 3 to 4 times. Serve each portion over 1 cup of rice.

Nutrition: Calories: 484; Fat: 13g; Protein: 31g; Carbs: 59g

28. Crispy Tofu and Chickpea Bowl
Preparation time: 10 minutes
Cooking time: 9-13 minutes
Servings: 4
Ingredients:
- 1 (14-oz) container of extra-firm tofu, drained
- Nonstick cooking spray
- ¼ cup soy sauce
- ¼ cup water
- 2 tbsp rice vinegar
- 2 tbsp honey
- 1 tbsp cornstarch
- 2 garlic cloves, minced
- 2 cups cooked chickpeas
- 2 cups finely chopped broccoli
- 4 cups cooked brown rice
- 4 scallions, both white & green parts, sliced
- Sesame seeds, for garnish

Directions:
1. Cut the tofu into 4 lengthwise slabs. Place them between several layers of paper towels and press to drain. Cut the tofu into ½-inch cubes.
2. Heat your large skillet over medium-high heat and coat it with cooking spray. Add the tofu and cook for 5 to 7 minutes, stirring regularly until browned.
3. Meanwhile, in a small bowl, mix the soy sauce, water, vinegar, honey, cornstarch, and garlic. Set aside.
4. Once the tofu is browned, add the chickpeas and broccoli, then sauté for 3 to 4 more minutes, until heated through.
5. Pour in the sauce and stir for 1 to 2 minutes until it thickens.
6. In each bowl, place 1 cup of rice. Divide the tofu and chickpea mixture between the bowls and drizzle with the sauce.
7. Garnish with the scallions and sprinkle with sesame seeds to serve.

Nutrition: Calories: 555; Fat: 10g; Protein: 26g; Carbs: 73g

29. Pork Souvlaki with Yogurt-Dill Dip

Preparation time: 15 minutes
Cooking time: 7 minutes
Servings: 4
Ingredients:

- 4 (4-oz) pork tenderloins, cut into 1-inch chunks
- 2 tbsp freshly squeezed lemon juice, divided
- ½ tbsp extra-virgin olive oil
- Sea salt & ground black pepper to taste
- ½ cup nonfat Greek yogurt
- ½ tbsp fresh dill
- ½ tsp minced fresh garlic
- 4 whole-wheat pitas

Directions:
1. Preheat a grill to high heat.
2. Toss the tenderloin chunks in 1½ tbsp lemon juice and oil in a large bowl. Season with salt and pepper.
3. Thread the chunks onto the skewers. Repeat with the remaining meat.
4. Grill the tenderloin skewers on all sides for 7 minutes, until the meat is pale and mostly white with mostly clear juices.
5. Remove the pork from your grill and let it rest for 3 to 5 minutes.
6. Meanwhile, mix the yogurt, dill, garlic, and remaining lemon juice in a medium bowl.
7. Remove the meat from the skewers and divide it equally among 4 pitas. Place 2½ tablespoons of yogurt-dill dip on top, and serve.

Nutrition: Calories: 436; Fat: 10g; Protein: 47g; Carbs: 40g

30. Tuna Power Wrap

Preparation time: 10 minutes
Cooking time: 0 minutes
Servings: 4
Ingredients:

- 2 (5-oz) cans of water-packed tuna, drained
- 4 extra-large hard-boiled eggs, peeled & chopped
- 4 celery stalks, finely chopped
- ½ cup nonfat plain Greek yogurt
- ½ cup chopped red onion
- 2 tsp whole-grain mustard
- Salt & ground black pepper
- 4 large whole-grain tortillas
- 1 cup alfalfa sprouts
- 2 small ripe tomatoes, sliced

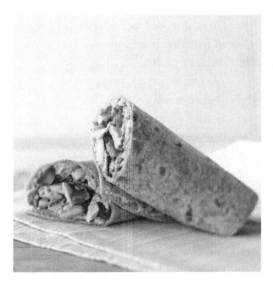

Directions:
1. In a large bowl, break apart the tuna. Mix in the eggs, celery, yogurt, onion, and mustard—season with salt and pepper.
2. Split the mixture between the tortillas and top with the alfalfa sprouts and tomatoes. Fold the sides in and roll the tortillas up.

Nutrition: Calories: 766; Fat: 24g; Protein: 64g; Carbs: 76g

31. Green Chicken Enchiladas

Preparation time: 10 minutes
Cooking time: 20 minutes

Servings: 6
Ingredients:

- 1 (15-oz) can of green enchilada sauce divided
- 12 corn tortillas
- 3 cups shredded rotisserie chicken
- 1 cup shredded cheddar cheese
- ½ cup nonfat plain Greek yogurt

Directions:

1. Preheat the oven to 350°F.
2. In a large casserole dish, pour about ¼ cup of the enchilada sauce and use a spoon to spread it out in the bottom of the dish.
3. Wrap the tortillas in your damp paper towel and heat in the microwave for 30 seconds or until pliable.
4. Place about ¼ cup of chicken in each tortilla and roll it up. Place the rolled tortillas in the prepared pan seam-side down.
5. Pour the remaining enchilada sauce over your tortillas. Top with the cheese.
6. Bake for 20 minutes, uncovered until the cheese is melted and bubbly.

Nutrition: Calories: 328; Fat: 12g; Protein: 26g; Carbs: 30g

32. Zucchini Pizza Boats

Preparation time: 15 minutes
Cooking time: 35 minutes
Servings: 3
Ingredients:

- 6 zucchini
- 1-pound lean ground beef
- ½ cup chopped onions
- Sea salt & ground black pepper to taste
- ¾ cup marinara pasta sauce
- ½ cup black beans
- ½ cup corn kernels
- ½ tsp dried basil
- ½ tsp dried oregano
- 1 cup grated cheddar cheese

Directions:

1. Preheat the oven to 375°F. Line a baking sheet with parchment paper.
2. Halve the zucchini lengthwise, then use a spoon to scoop out the insides so that about ½ inch of skin remains.
3. Put the scooped-out zucchini meat in a large bowl. Place the zucchini cut-side down on a cutting board to drain.
4. In your large skillet, cook the beef for 5 minutes over medium heat until only slightly pink inside.
5. Add the onions and cook for 3 minutes more until no pink is visible. Season with salt and pepper.
6. Put the beef and onions in the bowl with the scooped-out zucchini, and add the pasta sauce, black beans, corn, basil, and oregano.
7. Season with salt and pepper. Mix until well blended.
8. Turn the zucchini boats right-side up and place them on the lined baking sheet. Place the filling inside the zucchini boats, then top with the cheese.
9. Bake the zucchini for 25 minutes, then broil for about 2 more minutes until the cheese turns golden brown. Remove and let it cool. Serve.

Nutrition: Calories: 503; Fat: 29g; Protein: 39g; Carbs: 49g

33. Three-Bean Salad

Preparation time: 15 minutes
Cooking time: 0 minutes

Servings: 6
Ingredients:

- 1 (14-oz) can of kidney beans, drained & rinsed
- 1 (14-oz) can of chickpeas, drained & rinsed
- 1 (14-oz) can of white navy or cannellini beans, drained &
- rinsed
- ½ bunch of parsley, coarsely chopped
- 2 celery stalks, finely chopped
- 1 red bell pepper, finely chopped
- 1 jalapeño pepper, minced (optional)
- 1 garlic clove, minced (optional)
- ¼ cup apple cider vinegar
- ¼ cup extra-virgin olive oil
- 1 tbsp Dijon mustard
- 1 tbsp maple syrup
- ½ tsp salt
- Freshly ground black pepper to taste

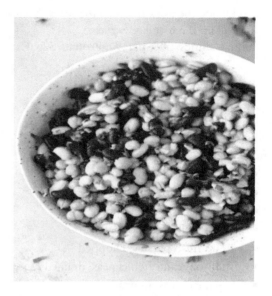

Directions:
1. In a medium bowl, combine the kidney beans, chickpeas, navy beans, parsley, celery, bell pepper, jalapeño pepper, and garlic (if using).
2. Add the apple cider vinegar, olive oil, mustard, maple syrup, salt, and pepper. Mix everything thoroughly, and serve.

Nutrition: Calories: 284; Fat: 10g; Protein: 11g; Carbs: 40g

34. Ginger-Hoisin Pork Wraps

Preparation time: 15 minutes
Cooking time: 11-13 minutes
Servings: 4
Ingredients:

- Nonstick cooking spray
- 1 yellow onion, diced
- 2 garlic cloves, minced
- 1 tsp minced ginger
- 1-pound lean ground pork
- 2 tbsp hoisin sauce
- 2 tbsp soy sauce
- 2 tbsp brown sugar
- 4 large whole-wheat tortillas
- 4 large lettuce leaves
- 2 carrots, shredded
- 1 red bell pepper, seeded & sliced
- 2 scallions, both white & green parts, sliced

Directions:
1. Heat your large skillet over medium heat and coat it with cooking spray.
2. Cook the onion for 5 minutes, until softened. Add the garlic and ginger, then cook for 30 seconds until fragrant.
3. Add the pork and cook for 5 to 6 minutes, until browned and cooked through.
4. Add the hoisin sauce, soy sauce, and brown sugar. Stir for 1 to 2 minutes more, until heated through and the pork is well coated. Turn off the heat.
5. On a clean work surface, lay the tortillas and top each with a lettuce leaf.

6. Divide the pork between the tortillas and top with the carrots, bell pepper, and scallions. Fold the sides in and roll up the tortillas. Serve.

Nutrition: Calories: 398; Fat: 9g; Protein: 32g; Carbs: 51g

35. Quinoa & Chickpea Tabboule

Preparation time: 20 minutes
Cooking time: 0 minutes
Servings: 6
Ingredients:
- 1 cup quinoa, cooked
- 1 cup tomato, chopped
- 1 cup cucumber, chopped
- 1 cup scallions, chopped
- 1 cup fresh parsley, chopped
- 1 (14-oz) can of chickpeas, drained & rinsed
- 2 garlic cloves, minced
- ¼ cup chopped mint
- 2 tbsp olive oil
- Juice of 1 lemon
- ½ tsp salt
- Freshly ground black pepper to taste

Directions:
1. Mix the quinoa, tomato, cucumber, scallions, parsley, chickpeas, garlic, and mint in your large bowl.
2. Pour the olive oil and lemon juice over the quinoa mixture, stirring in the salt and pepper. Serve immediately.

Nutrition: Calories: 170; Fat: 6g; Protein: 6g; Carbs: 25g

36. Lemon-Garlic Cod with Asparagus

Preparation time: 10 minutes
Cooking time: 15 minutes
Servings: 4
Ingredients:
- 1 pound cod fillets
- 1 lemon, zested and juiced
- 2 tsp extra-virgin olive oil, divided
- 3 garlic cloves, minced
- ½ tsp salt, divided
- ¼ tsp freshly ground black pepper
- 1 pound asparagus, trimmed
- ¼ cup chopped fresh parsley

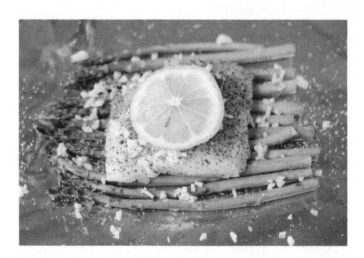

Directions:
1. Preheat the oven to 400°F.
2. On a large baking sheet, arrange the cod fillets. Sprinkle with the lemon zest and drizzle with the lemon juice and 1 tsp olive oil.
3. Season with the garlic, ¼ tsp salt, and pepper.
4. Arrange the asparagus around the cod and drizzle with the remaining 1 teaspoon of oil.
5. Bake within 12 to 14 minutes, until the cod flakes easily with a fork and the asparagus, is bright green and fork tender. Garnish with parsley and serve.

Nutrition: Calories: 137; Fat: 3g; Protein: 23g; Carbs: 6g

37. Feta Turkey Burgers

Preparation time: 15 minutes

Cooking time: 16 minutes
Servings: 4
Ingredients:

- 1 tbsp extra-virgin olive oil
- ½ medium onion, chopped
- 1 cup chopped baby spinach
- 2 garlic cloves, minced
- 1-pound lean ground turkey
- ½ cup crumbled feta cheese
- 2 tbsp chopped fresh basil
- 1 tsp dried oregano
- ½ tsp sea salt
- ¼ tsp freshly ground black pepper
- Nonstick cooking spray

Directions:

1. In your medium nonstick skillet over medium-high heat, heat the olive oil. Add the onion and sauté within 5 minutes or until translucent.
2. Add the spinach and garlic and sauté for 3 more minutes until the spinach is wilted.
3. Transfer to a large bowl and add the turkey, feta, basil, oregano, salt, and pepper.
4. Lightly spray the palms of your hands with nonstick spray, and use your hands to mix until well combined. Form into 4 equal-size patties.
5. Heat your large nonstick skillet over medium-high heat. Spray both sides of each patty lightly with the cooking spray, then place in the pan.
6. Cook for about 4 minutes on each side until cooked through. Serve.

Nutrition: Calories: 239; Fat: 14g; Protein: 27g; Carbs: 3g

38.Cauliflower Fried Rice

Preparation time: 15 minutes
Cooking time: 10 minutes
Servings: 6
Ingredients:

- 1 head cauliflower, cut into florets
- 1 tbsp sesame oil
- 1 white onion, finely chopped
- 1 large carrot, finely chopped
- 4 garlic cloves, minced
- 2 cups frozen edamame or peas
- 3 scallions, sliced
- 3 tbsp soy sauce
- Salt & ground black pepper to taste

Directions:

1. Process the cauliflower in your food processor until the cauliflower is the consistency of rice. Set aside.
2. Warm a large skillet over medium-high heat. Drizzle in the sesame oil and then add the onion and carrot for 5 minutes, until the carrots soften.
3. Stir in the garlic and cook within another minute. Add the cauliflower and edamame.
4. Heat for 5 minutes until the cauliflower softens. Add the scallions and soy sauce. Mix well—season with black pepper. Serve.

Nutrition: Calories: 117; Fat: 3g; Protein: 7g; Carbs: 19g

39.Ginger Beef Sirloin and Bok Choy

Preparation time: 10 minutes

Cooking time: 10 minutes
Servings: 4
Ingredients:

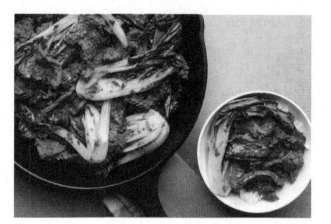

- 1 tbsp fresh ginger, minced
- 1 tsp garlic, minced
- ½ cup white onion, diced
- 1 pound beef sirloin, sliced against the grain into ¼-inch strips
- ½ tsp red pepper flakes
- ½ tsp ground cumin
- ½ tsp ground coriander
- 1 tbsp low sodium soy sauce
- 1 large Bok choy stalk, washed & sliced into ½-inch strips

Directions:
1. Generously spray a medium skillet with non-stick cooking spray and place over medium heat.
2. Add the ginger, garlic, and onion, and cook until the onions are soft, stirring frequently.
3. Adjust to medium-high heat and add the sirloin strips, red pepper flakes, cumin, and coriander.
4. Cook within 2 to 3 minutes or until the meat is browned. Add the soy sauce, and continue to cook for 1 to 2 minutes, stirring frequently.
5. Adjust to low heat. Add the Bok choy, cover, and steam for 5 minutes.
6. Remove the lid, and continue to cook on low for 2 to 3 minutes or until the liquid is reduced. Serve hot.

Nutrition: Calories: 242; Fat: 9g; Protein: 35g; Carbs: 3g

40. Steak-Spiced Tofu with Asparagus
Preparation time: 10 minutes
Cooking time: 30 minutes
Servings: 2
Ingredients:

- 1 (16-oz) package of extra-firm tofu
- 3 tbsp low-sodium steak spice
- 2 tbsp coconut oil, melted
- 1 bunch of asparagus, rough ends trimmed
- ½ lemon
- Salt & ground black pepper to taste
- Salsa or barbecue sauce (optional)

Directions:
1. Preheat the oven to 400°F. Line your baking sheet using parchment paper or a silicone liner.
2. Drain the water off the tofu, and then press the tofu with a hand towel to remove as much moisture as possible.
3. Slice your tofu in half horizontally, then slice each half horizontally again to make 4 steaks.
4. Place the tofu steaks on a baking sheet, leaving some room for the asparagus.
5. Whisk together the steak spice and oil in a small bowl to make a marinade.
6. Scoop out and rub the marinade over the tofu steaks, ensuring they are evenly coated on all sides.
7. Bake for 15 minutes. Remove from the oven and lay the asparagus on the steaks.
8. Squeeze the fresh lemon over the asparagus, then sprinkle with a few pinches of salt and pepper.
9. Return the sheet to the oven and bake for 15 minutes more. Remove from the oven and enjoy immediately.
10. Top the steaks with fresh salsa or your favourite barbecue sauce (if using).

Nutrition: Calories: 347; Fat: 27g; Protein: 25g; Carbs: 10g

Chapter 8. Dinner Recipes

41. Pork Chops with Mushroom Sauce
Preparation time: 10 minutes
Cooking time: 19-23 minutes
Servings: 4
Ingredients:

- 4 (3-oz) boneless pork chops
- 1 tsp salt
- ½ tsp paprika
- ¼ tsp) freshly ground black pepper
- 1 tsp avocado oil
- 8 oz sliced mushrooms
- 1 small yellow onion, julienned
- 3 garlic cloves, minced
- 2 tbsp all-purpose flour
- 1½ cups chicken broth
- ¼ cup low-fat cream
- 6 cups cooked brown rice

Directions:
1. Season the pork chops with salt, paprika, and pepper on both sides.
2. In your large skillet over medium-high heat, heat the oil. Sear the pork chops on each side for 3 to 4 minutes until golden brown.
3. Remove and set aside on a plate.
4. In your same skillet over medium heat, cook the mushrooms and onions for 5 minutes, until browned and the water is released and cooked out.
5. Add the garlic and cook within 30 seconds until fragrant.
6. Stir in the flour and mix well. Add the broth and let it simmer. Cook for 2 to 3 minutes until the sauce is thickened.
7. Add the cream and stir to heat through; then adjust to low heat.
8. Return the pork chops to your pan and cook for 6 to 8 more minutes, until the pork's juices clear. Serve over the rice.

Nutrition: Calories: 534; Fat: 8g; Protein: 29g; Carbs: 77g

42. Deconstructed Cabbage Roll Stew
Preparation time: 10 minutes
Cooking time: 35 minutes
Servings: 6
Ingredients:

- 1 tbsp olive oil
- 1 onion, chopped
- Pinch + ½ tsp salt, divided
- 2 garlic cloves, minced
- 2 cups brown mushrooms, chopped
- 1 cup brown lentils, dried
- 2 tsp thyme, dried
- 3 cups vegetable broth or water
- 1 (14-oz) can of diced tomatoes
- 1 small cabbage, coarsely chopped
- 2 tbsp apple cider vinegar
- Parsley, chopped, for garnish

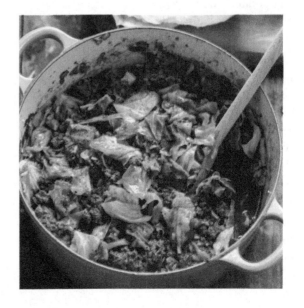

- 2 cups rice, cooked

Directions:

1. In your large stockpot, warm the oil over medium heat. Add the onion and salt.
2. Cook for 5 minutes until the onions become slightly translucent. Add the garlic and mushrooms and cook for about 5 minutes more until the mushrooms begin to release water.
3. Add the dried lentils, thyme, and broth or water, then let it boil. Adjust to low heat, cover, and simmer for 25 minutes or until the lentils have softened.
4. Stir in the tomatoes, cabbage, vinegar, and remaining salt and cook for 5 minutes more to allow the cabbage to soften.
5. Garnish with parsley and serve with rice.

Nutrition: Calories: 211; Fat: 3g; Protein: 10g; Carbs: 3g

43. Garlic Salmon, Sweet Potato, and Broccoli

Preparation time: 5 minutes
Cooking time: 25 minutes
Servings: 4
Ingredients:

- 1-pound frozen cubed sweet potatoes
- 1 tbsp extra-virgin olive oil, divided
- ½ tsp salt, divided
- ¼ tsp freshly ground black pepper, divided
- 1 tbsp maple syrup
- 1 tbsp whole-grain (or Dijon) mustard
- 2 garlic cloves, minced
- 8 oz chopped broccoli florets
- 20 oz salmon fillets

Directions:

1. Preheat the oven to 425°F. Line a baking sheet with parchment paper.
2. In your large bowl, toss the sweet potatoes with 1 tsp olive oil, ¼ tsp salt, and tsp pepper. Place them on the baking sheet and cook for 10 minutes.
3. Meanwhile, in a small bowl, mix 1 teaspoon of oil, maple syrup, mustard, and garlic.
4. Toss the broccoli with the remaining oil, salt, and pepper in the same large bowl.
5. After 10 minutes, remove the baking sheet from the oven and stir the sweet potatoes.
6. Arrange the broccoli and sweet potatoes around the edges and lay the salmon in the middle.
7. Spread the mustard sauce on the salmon and bake for 15 minutes, until the salmon flakes with a fork and the sweet potatoes are tender.

Nutrition: Calories: 322; Fat: 9g; Protein: 31g; Carbs: 29g

44. Adobo Sirloin Steak

Preparation time: 10 minutes
Cooking time: 8 minutes
Servings: 4
Ingredients:

- Juice of 1 lime
- 1 tbsp minced garlic
- 1 tsp dried oregano
- 1 tsp ground cumin
- 2 tbsp finely chopped canned chipotle chiles in adobo sauce + 2 tbsp sauce
- 4 (6-oz) sirloin steaks, trimmed of fat
- Salt & ground black pepper, to taste

Directions:

1. Add lime juice, garlic, oregano, cumin, chiles, and adobo sauce in your small bowl. Mix well to combine.
2. Season meat with salt and pepper. Place steaks into a large
3. Ziploc bag with adobo marinade.
4. Seal tightly and shake to coat. Refrigerate for at least 2 hours, shaking occasionally.
5. Prepare a grill to high heat. Lightly coat the grill grates with cooking spray.
6. Cook steaks for 4 to 5 minutes on each side until the desired doneness. Let the steaks rest for 10 minutes and serve.

Nutrition: Calories: 237; Fat: 6g; Protein: 39g; Carbs: 2g

45. Tofu & Veggie Tray Bake

Preparation time: 15 minutes
Cooking time: 35 minutes
Servings: 4
Ingredients:

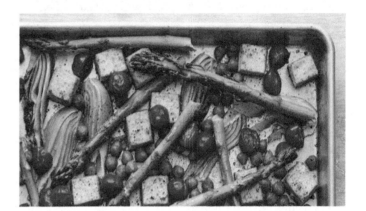

- 1 (16-oz) package of extra-firm tofu, chopped
- 4 cups cauliflower or broccoli, chopped
- 2 tbsp olive oil
- 1 tbsp nutritional yeast
- 1 tsp smoked paprika
- ½ tsp salt
- 1 bunch of asparagus, chopped, rough ends discarded
- 1-pint cherry tomatoes, halved

Directions:
1. Preheat the oven to 400°F. Line your baking sheet using parchment paper or a silicone liner.
2. Put the tofu and cauliflower in a large bowl. Pour in the oil, yeast, paprika, and salt. Mix until well combined.
3. Transfer the tofu and cauliflower to the baking sheet and bake for 20 minutes.
4. Remove the baking sheet and add the asparagus and tomatoes. Bake for 15 minutes more until the vegetables are tender.
5. Serve the tofu and veggies atop a bed of leafy greens with cooked rice or quinoa. Serve.

Nutrition: Calories: 231; Fat: 14g; Protein: 17g; Carbs: 15g

46. Lamb Shepherd's Pie

Preparation time: 10 minutes
Cooking time: 30 minutes
Servings: 4
Ingredients:

- 2 pounds Yukon gold potatoes, sliced into 1-inch pieces
- 1 tsp avocado oil
- ½ yellow onion, chopped
- 12 oz lean ground lamb
- 2 cups frozen carrots and peas
- 2 cups frozen cauliflower
- 2 tbsp whole-wheat flour
- ½ cup beef, chicken, or vegetable broth
- 1 tsp salt, divided
- ½ cup reduced-fat milk

Directions:
1. Preheat the oven to 350°F.
2. Fill your large pot with water and bring it to a boil over high heat. Add the potatoes and cook within 10 minutes, until tender.

3. Meanwhile, in a skillet over medium-high heat, heat the oil. Sauté the onion for 3 minutes, until beginning to soften.
4. Add the lamb and cook for about 5 minutes, until browned.
5. Add the carrots, peas, and cauliflower and cook for 5 more minutes, until heated through. Sprinkle with the flour and mix well.
6. Add the broth and ½ tsp salt and let it simmer for 1 to 2 minutes until thickening. Transfer the mixture to an 8-inch baking dish.
7. When the potatoes are done, drain and mash them with a potato masher. Add the milk and mix well—season with the remaining ½ teaspoon of salt.
8. Spread the potatoes on top of the lamb in an even layer. Bake for 5 minutes, until lightly browned. Serve.

Nutrition: Calories: 501; Fat: 20g; Protein: 25g; Carbs: 58g

47. Black Bean Quinoa Casserole

Preparation time: 10 minutes
Cooking time: 20 minutes
Servings: 6
Ingredients:

- 1 tbsp extra-virgin olive oil
- 1 medium red bell pepper, seeded & chopped
- 1 medium green bell pepper, seeded & chopped
- 1 large onion, chopped
- 6 cups cooked quinoa
- 4 (15- oz) cans of low-sodium black beans, drained & rinsed
- 1 (15-oz) can of diced tomatoes, drained
- 2 chipotles in adobo sauce, minced
- 2 cups low-fat shredded Mexican cheese blend

Directions:

1. Preheat the oven to 400°F.
2. In your large skillet over medium-high heat, heat the olive oil. Add the bell peppers and onion, then cook for 5 minutes, stirring, until the onions are softened.
3. In a large bowl, combine the quinoa, black beans, vegetable mixture, tomatoes, and chiles, and stir to combine.
4. Transfer the mixture to a large casserole dish and smooth the top. Sprinkle it with the cheese.
5. Bake for 15 minutes, until the cheese is melted and bubbly. Serve.

Nutrition: Calories: 710; Fat: 19g; Protein: 35g; Carbs: 72g

48. Dijon Mustard Baked Scallops

Preparation time: 5 minutes
Cooking time: 20 minutes
Servings: 1
Ingredients:

- 4 jumbo sea scallops (about 4 oz)
- 1½ tsp Dijon mustard
- 1½ tsp real maple syrup

Directions:

1. Preheat the oven to 350°F.
2. Place the scallops on a foil-lined baking sheet 1½ inches apart.
3. In a small bowl, mix the mustard and maple syrup. Spoon the mixture evenly over the scallops, and spread to coat the top.
4. Bake for 20 to 30 minutes until opaque. Serve warm.

Nutrition: Calories: 125; Fat: 1g; Protein: 17g; Carbs: 10g

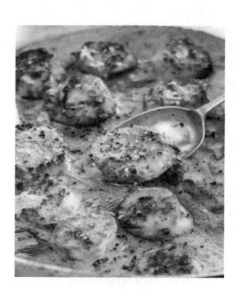

49. Flank Steak with Brussels Sprout

Preparation time: 5 minutes + marinating time
Cooking time: 16-18 minutes
Servings: 4
Ingredients:

- 6 tbsp) extra-virgin olive oil
- 1½ tbsp red wine vinegar
- 2 garlic cloves, minced
- 1½ tbsp honey
- ¾ tsp sea salt
- ¼ tsp freshly ground black pepper
- 1 pound flank steak, sliced into strips
- Nonstick cooking spray
- 1 pound Brussels sprouts, halved

Directions:

1. Whisk together the olive oil, vinegar, garlic, honey, salt, and pepper in your medium bowl.
2. Place the steak strips in a baking dish or bowl and top with two-thirds of the marinade. Cover and chill for an hour.
3. Spray a large sauté pan or skillet with cooking spray and heat over medium-high heat.
4. Add the Brussels sprouts and sauté for 8 to 10 minutes, stirring frequently, until lightly brown.
5. Pour the remaining marinade into the pan and cook until the Brussels sprouts are coated, and the sauce has reduced.
6. Divide the Brussels sprouts evenly among 4 plates.
7. Remove the steak from your marinade and place it in the pan over medium-high heat. Discard any extra marinade.
8. Pan fry for 4 minutes per side or until the steak is only slightly pink inside. Let cool.
9. Place 4 ounces of steak strips on each plate on top of the Brussels sprouts. Serve.

Nutrition: Calories: 477; Fat: 31g; Protein: 36g; Carbs: 17g

50. Baked Tamari Salmon and Zucchini

Preparation time: 5 minutes
Cooking time: 20 minutes
Servings: 4
Ingredients:

- 4 (6-oz each) salmon fillets
- 2 zucchini, halved lengthwise and sliced into ½-inch matchsticks
- ¼ cup tamari sauce
- 2 tbsp extra-virgin olive oil
- Sea salt & ground black pepper to taste

Directions:

1. Preheat the oven to 415°F.
2. Place the salmon fillets and zucchini slices on a baking sheet.
3. Mix the tamari sauce and oil in your small bowl, and brush it over the salmon and zucchini. Sprinkle with salt and pepper.
4. Bake within 15 to 18 minutes or until the salmon flakes apart when pierced with a fork. Remove from the oven and let cool.
5. Serve the zucchini with a salmon fillet.

Nutrition: Calories: 366; Fat: 20g; Protein: 42g; Carbs: 4g

51. Black Bean Burgers

Preparation time: 20 minutes + chilling time
Cooking time: 10 minutes

Servings: 8

Ingredients:

- 1 tbsp olive oil + extra for frying
- 1 cup sweet onion (such as Vidalia), finely chopped
- Pinch + ½ tsp salt, divided
- 4 garlic cloves, minced
- 2 (14-oz) cans of black beans, drained & rinsed
- ¾ cup chickpea flour
- ¼ cup vital wheat gluten
- ¼ cup fresh parsley, minced
- 1 tbsp oregano
- 1 tbsp smoked paprika

Directions:

1. In your large skillet, warm 1 tbsp oil over medium-high heat.
2. Add the onion and salt and sauté within a few minutes until the onions are soft. Add the garlic and cook within 1 minute more.
3. In your food processor, combine the cooked onions, garlic, half of the beans, chickpea flour, wheat gluten, parsley, oregano, remaining salt, and smoked paprika.
4. Pulse until the ingredients are well combined but slightly chunky.
5. Add in the remaining beans and pulse for about a minute, until chopped, but not fully processed.
6. Divide your mixture into 8 patties and place on a parchment-lined baking sheet. Transfer to the refrigerator to set for about 30 minutes.
7. Warm ½ tsp oil over medium-high heat in a large skillet. Add the burgers to the pan and cook for 5 minutes per side until browned. Serve wrapped in lettuce.

Nutrition: Calories: 143; Fat: 2g; Protein: 17g; Carbs: 14g

52. Spiced Pork Medallions with Apples

Preparation time: 15 minutes
Cooking time: 8-9 minutes
Servings: 4

Ingredients:

- 1 pound pork tenderloin, cut into 1-inch-thick medallions
- ½ tsp ground cumin
- ½ tsp garlic powder
- ½ tsp ground cinnamon
- ½ tsp salt
- ¼ tsp freshly ground black pepper
- 1 tbsp avocado oil
- 4 Granny Smith apples, cored & sliced
- 2 white onions, sliced

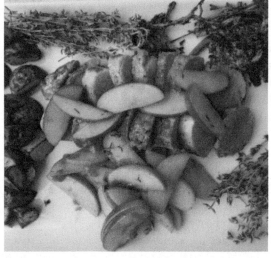

Directions:

1. Preheat the broiler on high.
2. Using a mallet, pound the medallions to ½-inch thick pieces. Rub with cumin, garlic powder, cinnamon, salt, and pepper.
3. Arrange on your baking sheet.
4. In your large skillet, heat the oil over medium-high. Sauté the apples and onions for 5 minutes, frequently stirring, until softened. Set aside.
5. Meanwhile, broil the pork on the oven rack closest to the broiler for 3 to 4 minutes per side, until the pork registers 145°F.
6. Serve the pork medallions topped with apples and onions.

Nutrition: Calories: 282; Fat: 5g; Protein: 27g; Carbs: 31g

53. Blackened Baked Tilapia Fillet

Preparation time: 20 minutes
Cooking time: 10-12 minutes
Servings: 5
Ingredients:

- 1 tbsp paprika
- 2 tsp dried thyme
- 1 tsp cumin
- 1 tsp dried oregano
- 1 tsp garlic powder
- 1 tsp onion powder
- 1 tsp salt
- ½ tsp ground black pepper
- ½ tsp red pepper flakes
- 2 pounds tilapia fillets (fresh or frozen)

Directions:

1. Preheat the oven to 400°F.
2. In your small bowl, combine the paprika, thyme, cumin, oregano, garlic powder, onion powder, salt, black pepper, and red pepper flakes.
3. Rinse the tilapia fillets and pat dry with a paper towel. Season both sides of your fillets with the rub, and let them sit at room temperature for 15 minutes.
4. Spray your 9 x 13-inch baking pan with nonstick cooking spray. Place the fillets in the pan and lightly spray the tops with the nonstick cooking spray.
5. Bake within 10 to 12 minutes or until the fish is firm and flaky. Serve hot.

Nutrition: Calories: 146; Fat: 3g; Protein: 32g; Carbs: 0g

54. Deconstructed Turkey Lasagna

Preparation time: 10 minutes
Cooking time: 20 minutes
Servings: 6
Ingredients:

- 20 oz extra-lean ground turkey
- ½ tsp salt, divided
- 8 oz wide egg noodles
- 3 cups store-bought marinara sauce
- ½ cup low-fat ricotta cheese
- ½ tsp garlic powder
- ¼ tsp freshly ground black pepper
- ½ cup shredded mozzarella cheese

Directions:

1. Preheat the oven to 350°F.
2. In your large skillet, crumble the turkey over medium-high heat and cook for 5 to 6 minutes, until cooked through. Season with a ¼ teaspoon of salt.
3. Meanwhile, boil a large pot of water and cook the noodles as stated in the package directions. Drain.
4. Once the turkey is cooked, add the marinara sauce and mix well. Let it simmer to heat through.
5. Combine the noodles, ricotta cheese, garlic powder, remaining salt, and pepper in a bowl.
6. Place half of the noodles in a large baking dish, then top with half of the meat sauce.
7. Add the remaining half of the noodles and then the remaining half of the meat sauce.
8. Top with the mozzarella cheese and bake for 10 minutes, until the cheese is melted.

Nutrition: Calories: 402; Fat: 9g; Protein: 40g; Carbs: 42g

55.Lentil and Zucchini Pasta Bake

Preparation time: 10 minutes

Cooking time: 20 minutes

Servings: 4

Ingredients:

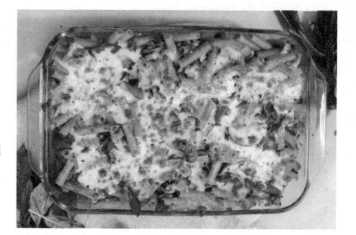

- 2 cups dry whole-grain pasta
- 2 tbsp extra-virgin olive oil
- 4 small zucchini, coarsely chopped
- 1 (8-oz) container of sliced mushrooms
- 1 large yellow onion, chopped
- 1 medium green bell pepper, seeded & chopped
- 2 (15- oz) cans of lentils, drained
- 1 (15-oz) can of diced tomatoes
- 1 cup reduced-fat cottage cheese
- ½ tsp dried oregano
- ½ tsp dried basil
- ½ tsp salt
- ¼ tsp freshly ground black pepper
- 1 cup shredded mozzarella cheese

Directions:

1. Preheat the oven to 350°F.
2. Boil your large pot of water over high heat and cook the pasta as stated in the package directions. Drain and set aside.
3. Meanwhile, in a skillet over medium-high heat, heat the oil. Sauté the zucchini, mushrooms, onion, and bell pepper for 10 minutes, until softened.
4. Add the lentils, tomatoes, their juice, cottage cheese, oregano, basil, salt, and pepper. Mix in the cooked pasta and transfer to a baking dish.
5. Cover with the mozzarella and bake for 10 minutes, until the cheese is melted. Serve.

Nutrition: Calories: 596; Fat: 13g; Protein: 36g; Carbs: 71g

56.Beef and Bean Chili

Preparation time: 10 minutes

Cooking time: 23 minutes

Servings: 4

Ingredients:

- 1 tsp avocado oil
- 1 (12-ounce) bag of frozen chopped onions and bell peppers
- 1 pound (453 grams) extra-lean ground beef
- 2 (15- oz) cans of black beans, drained and rinsed
- 1 (28-oz) can of crushed tomatoes
- 1 cup chicken stock
- ¼ cup tomato paste
- 2 tbsp chili powder
- ½ tsp salt
- ¼ tsp freshly ground black pepper

Directions:

1. In your large pot over medium-high heat, heat the oil. Add the frozen onions and peppers and cook for 3 minutes, until softened.
2. Add the beef and cook within 5 minutes until browned.
3. Stir in the black beans, tomatoes, chicken stock, tomato paste, chili powder, salt, and pepper.
4. Let it simmer, adjust to medium-low heat, and simmer for 15 minutes, until the flavors meld. Serve.

Nutrition: Calories: 349; Fat: 8g; Protein: 28g; Carbs: 44g

57. Shrimp Scampi with Whole-Grain Pasta

Preparation time: 10 minutes
Cooking time: 15 minutes
Servings: 4
Ingredients:

- 6 oz whole-grain linguini or spaghetti
- 2 tbsp extra-virgin olive oil
- 3 garlic cloves, minced
- 1 cup diced zucchini
- 12 oz shrimp, peeled & deveined
- 1 lemon, zested & juiced
- ½ cup shredded Parmesan cheese
- ½ cup chopped parsley

Directions:

1. Boil your large pot of water over high heat and cook the pasta as stated in the package directions until tender. Drain, reserving 1 cup of water.
2. Meanwhile, in your large skillet over medium heat, heat the oil. Add the garlic and cook within 30 seconds until fragrant.
3. Add the zucchini and cook for 3 to 4 minutes, until soft. Sauté the shrimp for 4 to 6 minutes, until pink and cooked through.
4. Turn off the heat and sprinkle the mixture with lemon zest and juice. Stir to combine.
5. Add the pasta to the skillet and stir to mix, adding about ½ cup of the reserved pasta water to create a loose sauce.
6. Add the remaining water, as needed, to coat the pasta. Sprinkle with the Parmesan and parsley, and serve.

Nutrition: Calories: 315; Fat: 12g; Protein: 23g; Carbs: 35g

58. Pork Meatball, Greens, and Beans Skillet

Preparation time: 10 minutes
Cooking time: 9 minutes
Servings: 4
Ingredients:

- 8 oz lean ground pork
- ¼ cup panko bread crumbs
- 1 large egg
- ¾ tsp salt, divided
- ¼ tsp freshly ground black pepper
- 1 tbsp avocado oil
- ½ cup chicken stock or water
- 8 cups collard greens, stems removed & roughly chopped
- 3 garlic cloves, minced
- 1 (15-oz) can of white beans, drained & rinsed

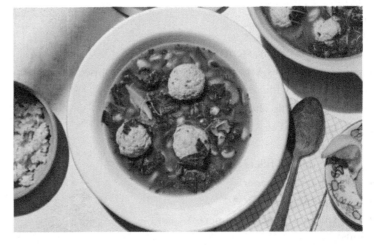

Directions:

1. In a small bowl, combine the pork, the bread crumbs, the egg, ½ tsp salt, and pepper.
2. Form the mixture into 16 small meatballs, each about 1 inch in diameter.
3. In your large skillet over medium-high heat, heat the oil. Cook the meatballs on each side for 1 to 2 minutes until browned. Transfer to a plate and set aside.
4. Add the chicken stock to your pan, scraping the bottom of the pan to release any cooked pieces.
5. Add the collard greens and garlic and stir until the greens are wilted.

6. Add the beans and the remaining salt and gently mix. Nestle the meatballs and any collected juices into the pan, cover, and cook for 5 more minutes until the juices run clear. Serve.

Nutrition: Calories: 252; Fat: 8g; Protein: 22g; Carbs: 24g

59. Mustard Almond-Crusted Chicken Breast

Preparation time: 10 minutes
Cooking time: 20-22 minutes
Servings: 4
Ingredients:

- ¼ cup liquid egg whites
- 3 tbsp Dijon mustard
- 1 cup almond flour
- ½ tsp paprika
- ½ tsp dried tarragon
- ½ tsp ground black pepper
- ½ tsp salt
- 1-pound chicken breasts, boneless, & skinless, cut into 2-inch strips

Directions:

1. Preheat the oven to 400°F. Line your large baking sheet using aluminium foil.
2. In your small bowl, whisk together the egg whites and mustard.
3. In a separate shallow baking dish, combine the almond flour, paprika, tarragon, black pepper, and salt.
4. Dip the chicken strips in the egg white mixture, then dredge in the almond flour mixture, making sure to coat the strips with the breading evenly.
5. Place the strips on the baking sheet. Bake within 20 to 22 minutes or until the juices run clear. Allow the chicken strips to rest for 5 minutes. Serve hot.

Nutrition: Calories: 278; Fat: 13g; Protein: 34g; Carbs: 5g

60. Cod Fillet with Charred Tomatillo Salsa

Preparation time: 10 minutes
Cooking time: 12 minutes
Servings: 2
Ingredients:

- 5 large tomatillos, stems & husks removed
- 2 serrano chiles, stems & seeds removed, chopped
- 2 tsp diced white onion
- ¼ cup roughly chopped fresh cilantro
- ½ tsp lime juice
- ½ tsp salt
- ½ pound cod fillets (fresh or frozen)
- ½ tsp garlic powder
- ½ tsp salt
- ½ tsp ground black pepper

Directions:

1. Preheat the broiler to low. Line a small baking pan with aluminium foil and place the tomatillos and serrano chiles in the pan.
2. Place the pan on the top oven rack and roast for 6 to 8 minutes, flipping the tomatillos and chiles halfway through the cooking process. Roast until nicely charred.
3. Add the tomatillos, chiles, onion, cilantro, lime juice, and salt to a blender. Pulse in 10-second intervals until a smooth consistency is achieved. Set aside.
4. Spray a small baking pan with nonstick cooking spray. Place the cod in the pan and season with the garlic powder, salt, and black pepper.

5. Broil for 3 to 4 minutes per side until the fish is lightly browned and can be flaked with a fork.

6. Transfer the baked cod to a serving platter and spoon the tomatillo salsa over the top. Serve hot.

Nutrition: Calories: 137; Fat: 1g; Protein: 25g; Carbs: 4g

61.Roasted Green Beans

Preparation time: 10 minutes
Cooking time: 15 minutes
Servings: 4
Ingredients:

- Nonstick cooking spray
- 1-pound fresh green beans, trimmed
- 3 garlic cloves, minced
- ¼ tsp salt
- ¼ tsp freshly ground black pepper

Directions:

1. Preheat the oven to 400°F. Line your large baking sheet with parchment paper and coat it with cooking spray.
2. Spread the beans onto the baking sheet and coat lightly with cooking spray.
3. Sprinkle with garlic, salt, and pepper. Toss well and arrange in one layer.
4. Cook for 15 minutes, stirring once about halfway through, until tender and browned in spots. Serve.

Nutrition: Calories: 39; Fat: 0g; Protein: 2g; Carbs: 9g

62.Sauteed Zucchini and Spinach

Preparation time: 10 minutes
Cooking time: 9-10 minutes
Servings: 6
Ingredients:

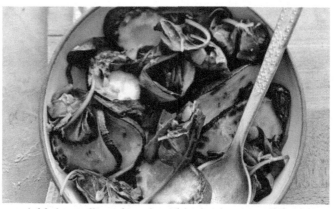

- 1 tbsp extra-virgin olive oil
- 2 cloves garlic, peeled & minced
- 2 zucchini, cut into matchsticks
- 2 cups grape tomatoes
- 3 cups baby spinach
- 1 tbsp lemon juice
- Pinch of ground black pepper

Directions:

1. Warm oil in a large pan over medium-low heat. Add the garlic and cook within 1 minute until fragrant.
2. Add the zucchini and adjust to medium heat. Cook for 3 to 4 minutes, stirring constantly.
3. Stir in tomatoes, cooking for 1 minute. Add the spinach, stirring and sautéing for another 3 to 4 minutes until wilted.
4. Add the lemon juice and black pepper before removing from the heat to serve.

Nutrition: Calories: 46; Fat: 2g; Protein: 2g; Carbs: 5g

63.Maple-Glazed Carrots

Preparation time: 5 minutes
Cooking time: 12-17 minutes
Servings: 4
Ingredients:

- 2½ pounds carrots, peeled & cut into 1-inch pieces
- 4 tbsp butter
- ¼ cup pure maple syrup
- 1 tbsp chopped fresh parsley
- Sea salt & ground black pepper to taste

Directions:

1. Fill your large saucepan halfway with water and let it boil over high heat. Salt the water.

2. Parboil the carrots in the salted water for about 2 minutes. Drain.
3. Wipe out the saucepan, melt the butter over medium heat, and sauté the carrots for 10 to 15 minutes until nearly tender.
4. Season it with salt and pepper, then add the maple syrup. Garnish with the parsley, and serve.

Nutrition: Calories: 266; Fat: 12g; Protein: 2g; Carbs: 40g

64. Thyme Roasted Turnips

Preparation time: 10 minutes
Cooking time: 20 minutes
Servings: 4
Ingredients:

- 1-pound large turnips, cut into 1-inch pieces
- 2 tsp extra-virgin olive oil
- 1 tsp dried thyme
- ½ tsp salt
- ¼ tsp freshly ground black pepper

Directions:
1. Preheat the oven to 400°F. Line your large baking sheet with parchment paper.
2. Drizzle the turnips on the prepared baking sheet with the olive oil and sprinkle with the thyme. Toss well. Sprinkle with salt and pepper.
3. Bake within 20 minutes, stirring once or twice, until tender and lightly browned. Serve.

Nutrition: Calories: 52; Fat: 2g; Protein: 1g; Carbs: 7g

65. Stir-Fried Asparagus and Mushroom

Preparation time: 5 minutes
Cooking time: 4 minutes
Servings: 3
Ingredients:

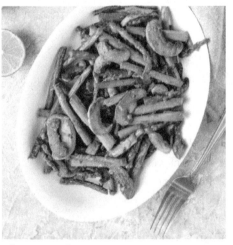

- 8 oz asparagus, trimmed & slice on the bias into 2-inch pieces
- 6 oz fresh shiitake mushrooms, stem removed & slice the caps into ½-inch slices
- 1 tbsp sesame oil
- 2 tsp minced fresh garlic
- 1 tsp peeled & minced fresh ginger
- Crushed red chilies

Directions:
1. Heat the sesame oil in your large sauté pan or skillet over medium-high heat. Add the garlic and ginger, then stir-fry for a few seconds.
2. Add the mushrooms and asparagus, and stir-fry for 1 minute.
3. Add the crushed chilies and stir-fry for 3 minutes until the asparagus is nearly tender. Let it cool, and serve.

Nutrition: Calories: 106; Fat: 5g; Protein: 4g; Carbs: 10g

66. Roasted Butternut Squash

Preparation time: 5 minutes
Cooking time: 25 minutes
Servings: 4
Ingredients:

- 1 (16-oz) bag of fresh chopped butternut squash
- 2 tsp extra-virgin olive oil
- ½ tsp salt

- ¼ tsp freshly ground black pepper

Directions:
1. Preheat the oven to 400°F. Line your large baking sheet with parchment paper.
2. Drizzle the squash with the olive oil on the prepared baking sheet and toss well. Sprinkle with salt and pepper.
3. Bake for 25 minutes, stirring once or twice until the squash is tender. Serve.

Nutrition: Calories: 66; Fat: 2g; Protein: 1g; Carbs: 12g

67.Smashed Sweet Potatoes

Preparation time: 5 minutes
Cooking time: 60 minutes
Servings: 6
Ingredients:

- 2 pounds sweet potatoes, washed & ends trimmed
- ½ cup light coconut milk
- 2 tsp ground cinnamon
- ½ tsp ground cayenne pepper

Directions:
1. Preheat the oven to 400°F. Pierce the sweet potatoes using a fork and individually wrap them in aluminum foil.
2. Place directly on your oven rack and bake for 1 hour, turning the potatoes halfway through the baking time.
3. Remove the potatoes and allow them to cool for 20 minutes. Once cooled, discard the foil and peel the skin from the potatoes.
4. In a large bowl, combine the peeled sweet potatoes, coconut milk, cinnamon, and cayenne pepper.
5. In your immersion blender, thoroughly smash the ingredients together until a smooth consistency is achieved. Serve warm.

Nutrition: Calories: 139; Fat: 1g; Protein: 2g; Carbs: 31g

68.Thyme-Cauliflower Purée

Preparation time: 10 minutes
Cooking time: 10 minutes
Servings: 6
Ingredients:

- 3 cups vegetable broth
- 2 medium cauliflower heads, chopped into florets
- 3 garlic cloves, minced
- 2 tbsp extra-virgin olive oil
- 2 tbsp coconut oil
- 1 tbsp chopped fresh thyme
- 1 tsp sea salt, + more for seasoning
- ¼ tsp freshly ground black pepper, + more for seasoning

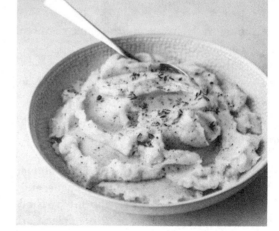

Directions:
1. Let the broth boil in your large stockpot and add the cauliflower. Adjust to a simmer for 10 minutes.
2. Remove the cauliflower from the heat and transfer it to a food processor.
3. Add the garlic, olive oil, coconut oil, thyme, salt, and pepper, and process until puréed.
4. Season with additional salt and pepper. Let it cool, and serve.

Nutrition: Calories: 150; Fat: 10g; Protein: 7g; Carbs: 12g

69.Honey-Glazed Brussels Sprouts

Preparation time: 10 minutes
Cooking time: 20 minutes
Servings: 4

Ingredients:

- Nonstick cooking spray
- 1 (9-oz) bag of shredded Brussels sprouts
- ½ tsp salt
- ¼ tsp freshly ground black pepper
- 2 tbsp maple syrup

Directions:

1. Preheat the oven to 400°F. Line your baking sheet with parchment paper and coat it with cooking spray.
2. Cut each half of the squash lengthwise, then cut each piece into ½-inch-thick strips.
3. In a bowl, toss the squash and Brussels sprouts and arrange them in a single layer on the baking sheet.
4. Coat lightly with cooking spray and sprinkle with salt and pepper. Mix well.
5. Cover the tray loosely with foil and bake for 10 minutes. Discard the foil, stir, and bake for 10 more minutes, until tender.
6. Drizzle with the maple syrup, toss and serve warm.

Nutrition: Calories: 129; Fat: 3g; Protein: 5g; Carbs: 24g

70.Sauté Garlicky Greens & Beans

Preparation time: 5 minutes
Cooking time: 10 minutes
Servings: 3
Ingredients:

- 2 tbsp extra-virgin or coconut oil
- 1 bunch of collards, stems & leaves chopped, separated
- 3 to 4 garlic cloves minced
- Pinch of salt
- 1 (14-oz) can of kidney beans, drained, rinsed, & dried
- Freshly ground black pepper to taste

Directions:

1. Warm the oil over medium heat in your large sauté pan or skillet. Add the collard stems, garlic, and salt.
2. Sauté for a few minutes until slightly golden. Add the collard leaves and continue to cook, stirring frequently.
3. Add a few splashes of apple cider vinegar or a squeeze of fresh lemon if needed to keep the pan moist.
4. After about 5 minutes, add the beans just to warm them up—season with salt and pepper. Serve.

Nutrition: Calories: 155; Fat: 10g; Protein: 6g; Carbs: 15g

71.Asparagus and Green Pea Salad
Preparation time: 15 minutes
Cooking time: 5 minutes
Servings: 4
Ingredients:

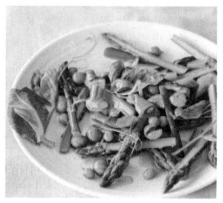

- 1 (16-oz) bag of frozen green peas
- 1 pound asparagus, trimmed & thinly cut on the bias
- 1 small red onion, halved & thinly sliced into half-moons
- 1 bunch of fresh mint, stems removed & leaves thinly sliced
- ¼ cup Balsamic Vinaigrette

Directions:
1. Boil your large pot of water over high heat. Add the peas and cook for 2 to 3 minutes, until bright green.
2. Drain and run under cold water to stop the cooking and chill the peas.
3. Toss the peas, asparagus, onion, mint, and vinaigrette in a large bowl. Serve.

Nutrition: Calories: 141; Fat: 2g; Protein: 9g; Carbs: 25g

72.Healthy Quinoa Salad
Preparation time: 5 minutes
Cooking time: 20 minutes
Servings: 4
Ingredients:

- 1 cup vegetable broth
- ½ cup quinoa, rinsed
- ½ red bell pepper, chopped
- ½ medium onion, chopped
- ¼ English cucumber, peeled, seeded, & chopped
- 2 tbsp finely chopped fresh mint
- Juice of ½ lime
- 2 tbsp extra-virgin olive oil
- Sea salt & ground black pepper to taste

Directions:
1. In a medium saucepan, boil the vegetable broth.
2. Add the quinoa, cover, and adjust to medium-low heat. Cook for 15 minutes or until all liquid is absorbed.
3. In a medium bowl, combine the quinoa, bell pepper, onion, cucumber, mint, lime juice, and olive oil. Season with salt and pepper, then mix well. Serve.

Nutrition: Calories: 165; Fat: 9g; Protein: 5g; Carbs: 16g

73.Tuna Bean Salad
Preparation time: 5 minutes
Cooking time: 0 minutes
Servings: 2
Ingredients:

- 4 cups blanched green beans
- 2 cups mixed cooked beans, rinsed & drained
- 1 cup frozen corn kernels, thawed
- 1 cup halved grape tomatoes
- 2 tbsp Dijon mustard
- 2 tbsp red wine vinegar

- Drizzle extra-virgin olive oil or avocado oil
- 1 (6-oz) can of flaked tuna, drained

Directions:

1. Mix the green beans, mixed beans, corn, tomatoes, mustard, and vinegar in a medium bowl. Drizzle with the olive oil and mix again.
2. Into each of 2 bowls, put half a can of tuna and 4 cups of bean salad. Serve.

Nutrition: Calories: 430; Fat: 6g; Protein: 38g; Carbs: 41g

74. Arugula Beets Salad

Preparation time: 10 minutes
Cooking time: 0 minutes
Servings: 3
Ingredients:

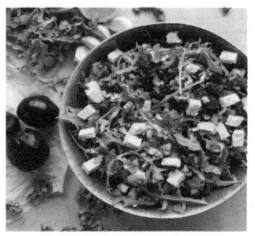

- 3 tbsp extra-virgin olive oil
- 3 tbsp freshly squeezed lemon juice
- 3 tbsp Dijon mustard
- 1 tbsp pure maple syrup
- 3 beets, peeled, chopped, & cooked
- 6 tbsp crumbled feta cheese, divided
- 6 tbsp walnut pieces, divided
- 9 cups arugula, divided

Directions:

1. Mix the olive oil, lemon juice, mustard, and maple syrup in your small bowl.
2. Into each of 3 jars, place a heaping 3 tbsp dressing topped by one-third of the chopped beets, 2 tbsp feta, 2 tbsp walnuts, and 3 cups of arugula. Seal.
3. To serve, shake the jar before opening it.

Nutrition: Calories: 346; Fat: 27g; Protein: 10g; Carbs: 20g

75. Bodybuilder Broccoli Salad

Preparation time: 10 minutes
Cooking time: 0 minutes
Servings: 4
Ingredients:

- 2 tbsp pure maple syrup
- 1 tbsp freshly squeezed lemon juice
- 2 to 3 tbsp light mayonnaise
- ½ cup nonfat plain Greek yogurt
- 1 broccoli head, finely chopped
- ¼ cup finely chopped red onion
- ¼ cup raw sunflower seeds
- ¼ cup dried cranberries
- ½ cup fresh blueberries

Directions:

1. Mix maple syrup, lemon juice, mayonnaise, and yogurt in your small bowl. Set aside.
2. In your large bowl, combine the broccoli, onion, sunflower seeds, cranberries, and blueberries. Add the dressing, and stir until well combined.
3. Divide the salad evenly among 4 bowls and serve.

Nutrition: Calories: 174; Fat: 8g; Protein: 6g; Carbs: 22g

76. Lentil Carrot Soup

Preparation time: 5 minutes

Cooking time: 20 minutes
Servings: 6
Ingredients:

- 2 tbsp extra-virgin olive oil
- 1 large onion, chopped
- 2 medium carrots, chopped
- 3 medium celery stalks, chopped
- 3 garlic cloves, minced
- 6 cups low-sodium vegetable broth or water
- 2 cups red lentils
- ½ tsp salt
- ¼ tsp freshly ground black pepper
- 2 cups chopped spinach
- 1 medium lemon, cut into wedges

Directions:

1. In your large pot over medium-high heat, heat the oil. Cook the onions, carrots, and celery for 5 minutes until they soften.
2. Add the garlic and cook within 30 seconds until fragrant.
3. Add the broth, lentils, salt, and pepper. Let it simmer and cook for 15 minutes until the lentils are tender.
4. Add the spinach and cook within 1 to 2 minutes until just wilted. Serve with a wedge of lemon.

Nutrition: Calories: 309; Fat: 6g; Protein: 17g; Carbs: 49g

77.Carrot and Spinach Soup

Preparation time: 10 minutes
Cooking time: 13 minutes
Servings: 4
Ingredients:

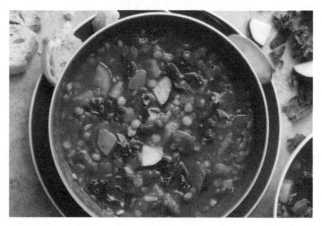

- 6 multicolored carrots, cut into 1-inch pieces
- ½ cup barley
- 1 (15-oz) can have diced tomatoes
- 2 garlic cloves, minced
- 4 cups of no-sodium vegetable broth
- 2 cups water
- 4 cups fresh spinach
- ¼ cup chopped fresh basil leaves, + more for garnish
- 2 tablespoons chopped fresh chives, + more for garnish
- 1 (15-oz) can of cannellini beans, rinsed & drained
- 1 tbsp balsamic vinegar
- Freshly ground black pepper, to taste

Directions:

1. In your large pot over medium heatcombine the carrots, barley, tomatoes with their juices, garlic, vegetable broth, and water. Let it simmer.
2. Cover the pot and cook for 10 minutes or until the barley is chewy and not hard.
3. Place spinach, basil, and chives on the water but do not stir. Cover the pot, adjust to low heat, and cook for 3 minutes to soften the leaves.
4. Stir the pot and add the cannellini beans and vinegar. Remove the pot and let it sit for 5 minutes, covered.
5. Garnish with chives, basil, and a pinch of pepper to serve.

Nutrition: Calories: 262; Fat: 2g; Protein: 12g; Carbs: 49g

78. Chicken Tortilla Soup

Preparation time: 5 minutes
Cooking time: 30 minutes
Servings: 4
Ingredients:

- 4 cups low-sodium chicken stock
- 1 tbsp avocado oil
- ½ medium white onion, diced small
- 1 garlic clove, minced
- ¼ jalapeño, seeded & minced
- 1 tomato, diced
- 1 cup cooked, diced chicken breast
- 1 tbsp freshly squeezed lime juice
- ¼ tsp dried oregano
- ⅛ tsp freshly ground black pepper

Directions:

1. In a medium stockpot, bring the chicken stock to a simmer.
2. In a large skillet, heat the avocado oil. Add the onion and sauté for about 3 to 4 minutes, until slightly tender.
3. Add the garlic and jalapeño, then sauté for another few minutes until softened.
4. Add the tomato to the skillet, and sauté for another 3 to 4 minutes, until tender.
5. Add the sautéed veggies, cooked chicken, lime juice, oregano, and pepper to the broth and simmer for 15 minutes. Remove from the heat and cool. Serve.

Nutrition: Calories: 104; Fat: 5g; Protein: 13g; Carbs: 2g

79. Split Pea Soup

Preparation time: 15 minutes
Cooking time: 50 minutes
Servings: 6
Ingredients:

- 2 tbsp olive oil
- 1 medium onion, coarsely chopped
- 2 carrots, coarsely chopped
- 2 celery stalks, coarsely chopped
- Pinch of salt, + 2 tsp, divided
- 2 cups yellow split peas, rinsed & drained
- 8 cups water
- 1 bay leaf
- 1 tsp paprika
- Freshly ground black pepper to taste
- 6 cups spinach, chopped

Directions:

1. In your large stockpot, warm the oil over medium heat. Add the onion, carrots, celery, and a pinch of salt, and cook until the onions soften.
2. Add the split peas, water, bay leaf, paprika, remaining salt, and pepper. Let it boil.
3. Once boiling, adjust to low heat and simmer for 50 minutes, occasionally stirring, until the split peas are soft.
4. Remove and discard the bay leaf. Stir in the spinach and sausage (if using) and cook for a couple of minutes more season with salt and pepper. Serve.

Nutrition: Calories: 362; Fat: 10g; Protein: 25g; Carbs: 46g

80. Turkey White Bean Soup

Preparation time: 10 minutes

Cooking time: 27 minutes
Servings: 4
Ingredients:

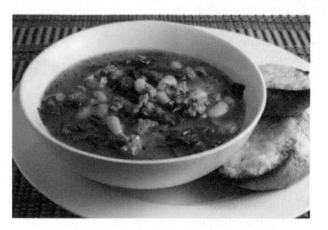

- 2 tsp extra-virgin olive oil
- 1 onion, chopped
- 1 clove garlic, minced
- 1¼ pounds lean turkey sausage, casings removed
- 6 cups low-sodium chicken broth
- 1 cup canned white beans, drained & rinsed
- 1 cup roughly chopped kale, stems removed
- Salt & ground black pepper, to taste

Directions:

1. In a medium heavy-duty pot, warm oil over medium-high heat. Add onion and garlic, sautéing for 2 to 3 minutes.
2. Add sausage, using a wooden spoon to break the meat into small pieces. Sauté for 5 to 6 minutes, stirring, until the meat is cooked.
3. Stir in chicken broth and beans. Cover with a lid and simmer for 10 minutes over low heat.
4. Add the kale and continue simmering with the pot covered for another 10 minutes.
5. Season with salt and pepper, and divide the soup into 4 bowls to serve.

Nutrition: Calories: 351; Fat: 15g; Protein: 34g; Carbs: 20g

81.Sweet Potato Nachos

Preparation time: 10 minutes
Cooking time: 40 minutes
Servings: 4
Ingredients:

- 3 small sweet potatoes, cut into ¼-inch rounds
- 1 cup black beans
- ½ cup cilantro, chopped
- 3 scallions, chopped
- ½ cup salsa
- 1 avocado, chopped
- 1 lime
- Salt to taste

Directions:

1. Preheat the oven to 400°F. Line your baking sheet using parchment paper or a silicone liner.
2. Spread the potatoes on the baking sheet in one layer.
3. Bake within 20 minutes, flip the potatoes and bake for 15 minutes more.
4. Remove the baking sheet and sprinkle the beans over the potatoes. Turn the oven to broil and cook the potatoes and beans for 5 minutes.
5. Remove from the oven and sprinkle with cilantro, scallions, salsa, and avocado. Squeeze some fresh lime on the nachos and sprinkle with salt. Serve.

Nutrition: Calories: 226; Fat: 7g; Protein: 7g; Carbs: 37g

82.Coconut-Cranberry Trail Mix

Preparation time: 5 minutes
Cooking time: 0 minutes
Servings: 4
Ingredients:

- 6 oz whole-grain pretzels
- 1 cup dried cranberries
- ½ cup coconut flakes
- ¼ cup shelled sunflower seeds
- ¼ cup raw almonds
- ¼ cup walnut pieces

Directions:

1. Combine the pretzels, cranberries, coconut, sunflower seeds, almonds, and walnuts in a bowl.
2. Mix well and store in your airtight container at room temperature.

Nutrition: Calories: 323; Fat: 14g; Protein: 7g; Carbs: 50g

83.Tofu Nori Wraps

Preparation time: 5 minutes
Cooking time: 0 minutes
Servings: 1
Ingredients:

- 1 (16-oz) package of extra-firm tofu
- 2 sheets of nori seaweed
- ¼ avocado, mashed
- ¼ cup brown or white rice, cooked
- ⅓ cucumber, cut into matchsticks

- 1 small package of sprouts or microgreens
- Soy sauce for serving

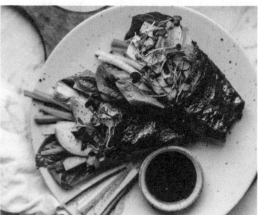

Directions:
1. Slice the tofu into pieces ¾ inch thick and 4 inches long. Set aside.
2. Place a sheet of nori, shiny side facedown and long side facing you, on a clean, dry cutting board.
3. Spread half of the mashed avocado evenly along the nori. Then cover the avocado with half of the rice.
4. Next, lay out 1 piece of tofu, half of the cucumber, and some microgreens on the rice.
5. Use both hands to roll the nori from the edge closest to you, slowly tucking and rolling to keep the filling in.
6. When you're just about to reach the end of your roll, dip your finger in a bit of water and dab the water along the edge of the nori to seal your roll (like an envelope). Set aside.
7. Repeat the process for the second nori sheet, and enjoy your rolls dipped in soy sauce.

Nutrition: Calories: 553; Fat: 29g; Protein: 51g; Carbs: 31g

84.Tuna Salad Rice Cakes

Preparation time: 5 minutes
Cooking time: 0 minutes
Servings: 2
Ingredients:
- 1 (6-oz) can of flaked tuna packed in water, drained
- 1 avocado, finely chopped
- ¼ red bell pepper, chopped
- 1 celery stalk, chopped
- ¼ red onion, chopped
- 1 lemon wedge, juiced
- Sea salt & ground black pepper to taste
- 4 rice cakes or 4 large romaine lettuce leaves

Directions:
1. Mix the tuna, avocado, bell pepper, celery, and onion in a medium bowl. Drizzle with lemon juice, then season it with salt and pepper.
2. To serve, spread on the rice cakes or serve wrapped in 2 lettuce leaves.

Nutrition: Calories: 332; Fat: 16g; Protein: 28g; Carbs: 25g

85.Apple Cinnamon Stacks

Preparation time: 5 minutes
Cooking time: 0 minutes
Servings: 1
Ingredients:
- 1 apple, skin on, cored, & cut crosswise
- ¼ cup peanut butter or nut or seed butter
- Pinch of cinnamon

Directions:
1. Lay out half of the apple slices on a cutting board and spread a bit of peanut butter and a sprinkling of cinnamon on them.
2. Place the other half of the apple slices on top of the peanut butter to make mini apple sandwiches.

Nutrition: Calories: 496; Fat: 33g; Protein: 17g; Carbs: 44g

86.Endive Hummus & Hemp Boats

Preparation time: 5 minutes

Cooking time: 0 minutes

Servings: 1

Ingredients:

- 1 endive, bottom ½ inch trimmed off, leaves removed
- ½ cup store-bought hummus
- 2 tbsp hemp hearts

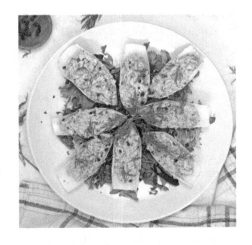

Directions:

1. Fill each endive spear with about 1 tablespoon of hummus.
2. Then sprinkle hemp hearts on top of the hummus. Serve immediately.

Nutrition: Calories: 421; Fat: 26g; Protein: 23g; Carbs: 30g

87.Tofu Chili Fries

Preparation time: 5 minutes

Cooking time: 40 minutes

Servings: 6 cups

Ingredients:

- 1 (16-oz) package of extra-firm tofu
- 2 tbsp coconut oil, melted
- 1 tbsp chili powder
- ½ tbsp oregano
- ½ tbsp basil
- ½ tsp salt
- ¼ tsp turmeric
- ¼ tsp onion powder
- ¼ tsp garlic powder
- Freshly ground black pepper to taste

Directions:

1. Preheat the oven to 400°F. Line your baking sheet using parchment paper or a silicone liner.
2. Remove excess moisture from the tofu by wiping it with a hand towel or paper towel.
3. Then slice it into fry-size pieces and transfer them to a shallow baking dish.
4. Mix the melted coconut oil, chili powder, oregano, basil, salt, turmeric, onion powder, garlic powder, and black pepper in a small bowl.
5. Pour the oil mixture over the tofu fries and ensure that the tofu pieces are evenly coated with the oil and spices.
6. Transfer the tofu fries to the lined baking sheet. Lay the pieces of tofu out with a bit of space in between.
7. Bake the fries for 20 minutes; then flip them and bake for 20 minutes until crispy. Serve.

Nutrition: Calories: 121; Fat: 9g; Protein: 9g; Carbs: 2g

88.Stuffed Avocado

Preparation time: 10 minutes

Cooking time: 0 minutes

Servings: 2

Ingredients:

- 1 (15- oz) can of black beans, drained & rinsed
- 1 (15-oz) can of sweet corn, drained
- 1 Roma tomato, diced
- 2 tbsp chopped cilantro
- Juice of 1 lime
- 1 garlic clove, minced

- Pinch of salt & ground black pepper
- 1 small avocado, halved & pitted

Directions:

1. Mix the black beans, corn, tomato, and cilantro in a small bowl. Add the lime juice and garlic, then season with salt and pepper.
2. Divide the bean salad between the avocado halves and serve.

Nutrition: Calories: 449; Fat: 14g; Protein: 17g; Carbs: 71g

89. Cinnamon-Roasted Chickpeas

Preparation time: 10 minutes

Cooking time: 45 minutes

Servings: 1 ½ cups

Ingredients:

- 1 (14-oz) can of chickpeas, drained, rinsed, & dried
- 1 tbsp maple syrup
- ½ tbsp olive oil
- ½ tsp cinnamon
- Pinch of salt

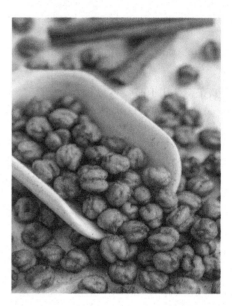

Directions:

1. Preheat the oven to 375°F. Line your baking sheet using parchment paper or a silicone liner.
2. Mix chickpeas, syrup, oil, cinnamon, and salt in a medium bowl. Spread the chickpeas on your baking sheet in one layer.
3. Bake for 20 minutes and then shake the baking sheet. Continue baking within 20 minutes more or until the chickpeas are crispy. Serve.

Nutrition: Calories: 173; Fat: 5g; Protein: 7g; Carbs: 27g

90. Smoky Tofu Bites

Preparation time: 10 minutes

Cooking time: 30 minutes

Servings: 4

Ingredients:

- 1 (12-oz) package of firm tofu
- 1 tbsp soy sauce
- 1 tsp extra-virgin olive oil (optional)
- ¼ tsp garlic powder
- ¼ tsp onion powder
- ¼ tsp smoked paprika

Directions:

1. Preheat the oven to 400°F. Line a baking sheet with parchment paper.
2. Drain the excess water off the tofu, pat it with a paper towel to dry, and then cut it into cubes.
3. Transfer the tofu cubes, soy sauce, oil, garlic powder, onion powder, and smoked paprika to a large bowl.
4. Mix until well combined and let it rest for at least 5 minutes.
5. Place the tofu cubes onto a baking sheet. Bake for 15 minutes, flip each of the tofu cubes and bake for 15 minutes more or until golden brown.

Nutrition: Calories: 74; Fat: 5g; Protein: 8g; Carbs: 2g

91. Pb & Banana Collard Green Wraps

Preparation time: 5 minutes

Cooking time: 0 minutes

Servings: 1
Ingredients:
- 1 large collard green leaf
- 1 banana, peeled
- 2 tbsp peanut butter

Directions:
1. Lay the collard green leaf out on a cutting board and spread peanut butter on top.
2. Add the banana and roll it up with the collard leaves. Serve.

Nutrition: Calories: 318; Fat: 17g; Protein: 11g; Carbs: 38g

92.High-Protein Crab Balls
Preparation time: 10 minutes
Cooking time: 20 minutes
Servings: 4
Ingredients:

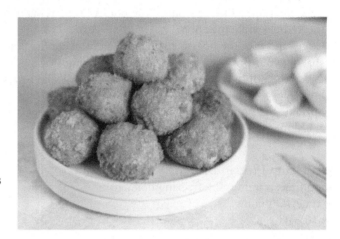

- Nonstick cooking spray
- 1 pound crab meat
- 1 cup panko bread crumbs
- 1 large egg, beaten
- 2 tbsp lemon juice
- 1 scallion, sliced, both white and green parts
- ½ tsp Old Bay seasoning
- ¼ tsp freshly ground black pepper

Directions:
1. Preheat the oven to 375°F. Line your baking sheet with parchment paper and coat it with cooking spray.
2. Mix the crab, bread crumbs, egg, lemon juice, scallion, Old Bay seasoning, and pepper in a small bowl.
3. Form the mixture into 12 balls, place them on the prepared baking sheet, and coat lightly with cooking spray.
4. Bake for 20 minutes, until lightly browned. Serve warm.

Nutrition: Calories: 184; Fat: 2g; Protein: 24g; Carbs: 17g

93.Bacon-Flavored Coconut Chips
Preparation time: 5 minutes
Cooking time: 12 minutes
Servings: 8
Ingredients:
- 2½ cups unsweetened coconut flakes, large
- 2 tbsp soy sauce
- 1 tbsp maple syrup
- 1 tsp liquid smoke

Directions:
1. Preheat the oven to 350°F. Line your baking sheet using parchment paper or a silicone liner.
2. Mix the coconut flakes, soy sauce, maple syrup, and liquid smoke in your medium bowl until everything is evenly coated.
3. Spread out the coconut flakes evenly on the baking sheet. Transfer the baking sheet to your oven and bake for 7 minutes. Stir the flakes to ensure they bake evenly.
4. Return to the oven and bake for 5 minutes more or until the coconut flakes are crispy.
5. Remove from the oven and transfer the chips to a container immediately to avoid overcooking.

Nutrition: Calories: 43; Fat: 3g; Protein: 1g; Carbs: 3g

94.Turmeric Popcorn
Preparation time: 5 minutes

Cooking time: 15 minutes
Servings: 6
Ingredients:

- 2 tbsp coconut oil
- ½ cup organic popcorn kernels
- ½ tsp turmeric
- 2 tbsp nutritional yeast
- Salt & ground black pepper to taste

Directions:

1. Warm a large stockpot over medium heat. Put the coconut oil and 3 popcorn kernels in the pot. Cover and cook until all 3 kernels pop.
2. Take the popped kernels out of the pot. Add the remaining popcorn kernels and shake the pot a bit to space the kernels while they pop.
3. Cover and take the pot off the heat. Wait 30 seconds. Put the pot back on the heat. Cook for 2 minutes, shaking your pot occasionally until the popping slows down.
4. When the popping has stopped, remove the pot's lid to release the steam; then transfer the popcorn to a big bowl.
5. Sprinkle the popcorn with turmeric and nutritional yeast, and season with salt and pepper. Serve.

Nutrition: Calories: 129; Fat: 8g; Protein: 4g; Carbs: 12g

95. Vanilla Hemp Protein Bars

Preparation time: 5 minutes + freezing time
Cooking time: 0 minutes
Servings: 16 bars
Ingredients:

- 2 cups Medjool dates, pitted
- 1 cup hemp hearts
- ½ cup vanilla protein powder
- ½ cup tahini

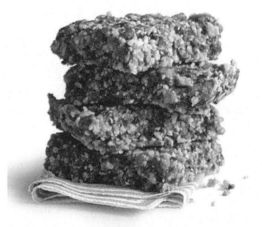

Directions:

1. In your food processor, pulse the dates until they are very well chopped (they may form a ball).
2. Add the hemp hearts, protein powder, and tahini, processing until evenly blended.
3. Line an 8-by-8-inch baking dish with parchment paper or a silicone liner. Transfer the dough to the baking dish.
4. Distribute the dough evenly and press it down with your hands. Transfer the baking dish to the freezer and let it set within 1 hour.
5. Remove from the freezer and slice into 8 large or 16 small bars.

Nutrition: Calories: 343; Fat: 19g; Protein: 17g; Carbs: 37g

96.Blueberry Cheesecake Cup

Preparation time: 10 minutes
Cooking time: 0 minutes
Servings: 4
Ingredients:

- For the crust:
- ⅔ cup graham cracker crumbs
- 2 tbsp coconut oil
- For the cheesecake filling:
- 1 cup nonfat vanilla Greek yogurt
- 1 cup low-fat cream cheese
- 1 tbsp honey
- 2 tsp freshly squeezed lemon juice
- 1 cup fresh blueberries, divided
- 2 tbsp crushed pecans, divided

Directions:

1. In your small bowl, stir the graham cracker crumbs and coconut oil.
2. In 4 round, airtight storage containers, place about 2½ tablespoons of the graham cracker crumbs and pack down using a spoon—place in the freezer to firm up.
3. Mix the yogurt, cream cheese, honey, and lemon juice in your stand mixer bowl until smooth and creamy.
4. Remove the crust containers from the freezer, and add about ¼ cup of the cream cheese filling to each.
5. Smooth with a spoon, then top each with ¼ cup of fresh blueberries and ½ tbsp crushed pecans. Serve.

Nutrition: Calories: 257; Fat: 10g; Protein: 14g; Carbs: 30g

97.Chocolate Banana Nice Cream

Preparation time: 5 minutes
Cooking time: 5 minutes
Servings: 4
Ingredients:

- 4 frozen bananas, chopped
- ¼ cup cocoa powder
- ¼ cup almond milk
- 1 (1 oz) scoop of chocolate protein powder

Directions:

1. In your food processor or high-speed blender, combine the frozen bananas, cocoa powder, milk, and protein powder.
2. Process until completely smooth and creamy. Serve.

Nutrition: Calories: 150; Fat: 2g; Protein: 7g; Carbs: 31g

98.Almond Butter Protein Bites

Preparation time: 15 minutes
Cooking time: 0 minutes
Servings: 24 protein bites
Ingredients:

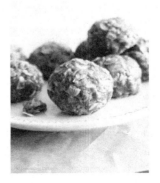

- ½ cup pitted dates
- ½ cup maple syrup
- ¼ cup almond butter
- ¼ cup ground flaxseed

- 2 scoops whey protein powder
- 1 cup rolled oats
- 2 tbsp dark chocolate chips

Directions:
1. In a food processor, combine the dates, maple syrup, almond butter, flaxseed, and whey and pulse to combine and break up the dates.
2. Add the oats and pulse until the dates are finely chopped. Stir in the chocolate chips.
3. Shape the mixture into 24 balls, about 1 inch in diameter. Serve.

Nutrition: Calories: 160; Fat: 5g; Protein: 7g; Carbs: 22g

99. Cocoa-Cranberry Energy Balls

Preparation time: 10 minutes
Cooking time: 0 minutes
Servings: 20 balls
Ingredients:
- ¼ cup almond butter
- 3 tbsp cocoa powder
- 2 tbsp coconut oil
- 2 tbsp honey
- ½ cup unsweetened shredded coconut, divided
- ¼ cup sunflower seeds
- ¼ cup hempseeds
- ¼ cup pecans
- ¼ cup dried cranberries
- Pinch of sea salt

Directions:
1. In your medium bowl, combine the almond butter, cocoa powder, coconut oil, and honey. Set aside.
2. In your food processor, combine ¼ cup of coconut with the sunflower seeds, hemp seeds, pecans, cranberries, and salt.
3. Pulse a few times until they are a coarse meal. Transfer the mixture to your bowl with the other ingredients and mix by hand until the dough sticks together, then shape it into 20 (1¼-inch) balls.
4. In a shallow bowl, place the remaining ¼ cup of coconut and roll the balls in the shredded coconut until well covered. Serve.

Nutrition: Calories: 208; Fat: 18g; Protein: 4g; Carbs: 9g

100. Black Bean Brownie Mug Cake

Preparation time: 5 minutes
Cooking time: 1 minute
Servings: 2
Ingredients:
- 1 tbsp chia seeds
- 3 tbsp water
- ½ cup cooked black beans
- 2 tbsp oat or whole wheat flour
- 2 tbsp cocoa powder
- 2 tbsp maple syrup
- 2 tbsp unsweetened almond milk
- ¼ tsp vanilla
- ⅛ tsp baking powder
- Pinch of salt

Directions:

1. Mix the chia seeds and water in your small bowl and set aside for at least 5 minutes.
2. In a small blender, combine the beans, flour, cocoa powder, syrup, milk, vanilla, baking powder, salt, and chia water mixture.
3. Process until the mixture resembles a smooth, batter-like consistency. Transfer equal parts of the batter to two microwave-safe mugs.
4. Microwave on high for 1 minute. Remove the mugs from the microwave and allow them to cool for 5 minutes. Serve.

Nutrition: Calories: 94; Fat: 2g; Protein: 3g; Carbs: 18g

101. Protein-Packed Rice Pudding

Preparation time: 5 minutes
Cooking time: 40 minutes
Servings: 4
Ingredients:

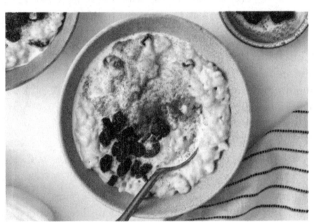

- 1 cup white rice
- 2½ cups unsweetened almond milk, divided
- 1 tsp vanilla extract
- 1 tsp cinnamon
- Pinch of salt
- ½ cup raisins
- 2 (1 oz) scoops vanilla protein powder

Directions :
1. In a small saucepan, combine the rice, 2 cups of almond milk, vanilla extract, cinnamon, and a pinch of salt.
2. Let it boil, cover, reduce the heat, and simmer within 35 minutes or until the rice is soft and the liquid is absorbed.
3. Stir in the raisins, protein powder, and remaining almond milk. Serve.

Nutrition: Calories: 329; Fat: 5g; Protein: 14g; Carbs:

102. Broiled Grapefruit with Yogurt

Preparation time: 5 minutes
Cooking time: 10 minutes
Servings: 2
Ingredients:

- 2 grapefruit, halved
- 4 tbsp packed brown sugar
- 2 cups nonfat plain Greek yogurt
- ¼ cup pecan pieces
- 2 tbsp honey

Directions:
1. Preheat the broiler on high.
2. Place the grapefruit, cut-side up, on a baking sheet and sprinkle each half with 1 tablespoon of brown sugar.
3. Broil for about 10 minutes until the sugar caramelizes and is bubbling.
4. Top each half with ½ cup yogurt, 1 tbsp pecan pieces, and ½ tbsp honey. Serve warm.

Nutrition: Calories: 515; Fat: 11g; Protein: 28g; Carbs: 82g

103. Pineapple Spice Sorbet

Preparation time: 5 minutes + freezing overnight
Cooking time: 0 minutes
Servings: 4
Ingredients:

- 1 pineapple, peeled, cored, & chopped
- 1 lime juice
- 1 piece of ginger, minced
- ⅓ cup coconut sugar
- ⅛ cup fresh basil leaves

Directions:
1. Add the pineapple, lime juice, ginger, coconut sugar, and basil leaves to a blender. Blend on a high speed. The consistency should be smooth.
2. Pour the smoothie mixture into a container, cover it with an airtight lid, and place it in the freezer overnight.
3. Before serving, remove the sorbet container from the refrigerator, and allow it to defrost slightly before serving.

Nutrition: Calories: 145; Fat: 0g; Protein: 1g; Carbs: 33g

104. Chocolate Peanut Butter Cups

Preparation time: 10 minutes + chilling time
Cooking time: 1-2 minutes
Servings: 12 peanut butter cups
Ingredients:

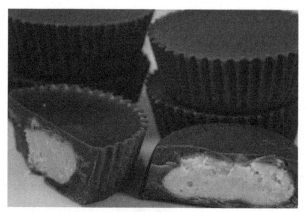

- 1 cup dark chocolate chips
- 1 cup peanut butter powder
- ¾ cup water

Directions:
1. Line a 12-cup muffin tin with ridged silicone liners.
2. In a microwave-safe bowl, heat the chocolate chips in 30-second intervals until melted, stirring between intervals.
3. Spoon about 2 teaspoons of chocolate into each cup.
4. Mix the peanut butter powder and water until smooth in your small bowl. Divide the mixture between the cups, about 1 tablespoon in each.
5. Reheat the remaining chocolate in the microwave until smooth and melted. Top each cup with the remaining melted chocolate, about 2 teaspoons each.
6. Place the cups in the refrigerator for about 15 minutes to set. Serve.

Nutrition: Calories: 121; Fat: 7g; Protein: 4g; Carbs: 11g

105. Very Berry Ice Cream

Preparation time: 5 minutes
Cooking time: 0 minutes
Servings: 5
Ingredients:

- 3 large, frozen bananas, chopped
- 1 tbsp almond butter
- ½ cup frozen sliced strawberries
- ¼ cup nonfat Greek yogurt
- 2 tbsp unsweetened vanilla cashew or almond milk

Directions:
1. Combine the bananas, almond butter, strawberries, yogurt, and cashew milk in a blender. Blend until well mixed.
2. In 5 freezer-safe storage containers, place ½ cup of ice cream and seal.

Nutrition: Calories: 126; Fat: 2g; Protein: 3g; Carbs: 27g

106. Poached Caramel Peache

Preparation time: 5 minutes

Cooking time: 9 minutes
Servings: 4
Ingredients:

- 2 cups of boiled water
- 1 cup of caster sugar
- 3 ripe peaches
- 1 lemon juice & zest
- ⅓ cup of blueberries
- 1 vanilla pod, cut in half, remove seeds

Directions:
1. Heat a small pan over medium heat, and caramelize the caster sugar. Swirl the sauce around in the pan without stirring it.
2. Add 2 cups of boiled water to the pan, and stir to combine, ensuring the sugar is dissolved.
3. Add the lemon zest and vanilla pod, then cook for 5 minutes.
4. Cut your peaches in half, and remove the pits. Add the peaches to the syrup, and let it simmer. Cook for 4 minutes, then switch off the heat.
5. Add the lemon juice to the pan and allow everything to cool down.
6. Divide the poached peaches into 4 glass mason jars, and add blueberries on top. Serve.

Nutrition: Calories: 360; Fat: 1g; Protein: 1g; Carbs: 94g

107. Lemon Drop Energy Balls

Preparation time: 10 minutes
Cooking time: 0 minutes
Servings: 12-14 balls
Ingredients:

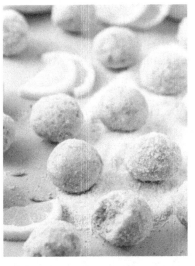

- 1¼ cups raw cashews
- 10 Medjool dates, pitted
- ½ cup shredded, unsweetened coconut, divided
- 1 tbsp coconut oil
- Zest of 1 lemon
- 1 tbsp freshly squeezed lemon juice

Directions:
1. In a food processor, process the cashews until roughly ground so that only tiny pieces remain. Remove from the food processor and set aside.
2. In the food processor, combine the dates, ¼ cup of coconut, coconut oil, and lemon zest until the dates are mashed.
3. Add the ground cashews and lemon juice, and process until a ball of dough starts to form.
4. Remove the dough from your food processor and, with your hands, roll it into 1½-inch balls.
5. In a shallow bowl, place the remaining coconut and roll the balls in the shredded coconut until well covered. Serve.

Nutrition: Calories: 265; Fat: 14g; Protein: 5g; Carbs: 35g

108. Blueberry PB Muffins

Preparation time: 10 minutes
Cooking time: 20 minutes
Servings: 12 muffins
Ingredients:

- Nonstick cooking spray
- 1 cup nonfat plain Greek yogurt
- ½ cup unsweetened applesauce
- ⅓ cup maple syrup

- ¼ cup skim milk
- 2 tbsp avocado oil
- 2 large eggs
- 2 cups oat flour
- ¼ cup peanut butter powder
- 1 tsp baking powder
- 1 cup fresh or frozen blueberries

Directions:
1. Preheat the oven to 350°F. Line a 12-cup muffin tin with ridged silicone liners.
2. In a large bowl, combine the yogurt, applesauce, maple syrup, milk, oil, and eggs.
3. Add the oat flour, peanut butter powder, and baking powder, and mix well.
4. Fold in the blueberries. Spoon the batter evenly into your muffin tin. Bake within 20 minutes until a toothpick inserted in the center comes out clean.

Nutrition: Calories: 167; Fat: 5g; Protein: 7g; Carbs: 24g

109. Vanilla Almond Truffles
Preparation time: 10 minutes
Cooking time: 0 minutes
Servings: 10-12 truffles
Ingredients:
- ½ cup smooth almond butter
- 3 tbsp maple syrup
- 1 tsp vanilla extract
- Pinch of salt
- ½ cup vanilla protein powder
- 1 tsp water, + more if needed

Directions:
1. Mix the almond butter, syrup, vanilla, and a pinch of salt in your medium bowl. Stir until well combined.
2. Stir in the protein powder. If it's a bit dry and crumbly, add in water 1 teaspoon at a time, and mix again until the mixture comes together nicely.
3. Roll out the truffles with about 1 tablespoon of mixture at a time. Use your hands to form the truffles.

Nutrition: Calories: 103; Fat: 7g; Protein: 4g; Carbs: 7g

110. Chickpea Choco Cookie Dough
Preparation time: 5 minutes
Cooking time: 5 minutes
Servings: 4
Ingredients:

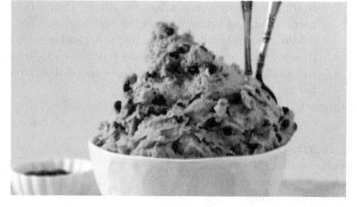

- 1½ cups chickpeas
- ¼ cup peanut butter or other nut butter
- 3 tbsp maple syrup
- 1 tsp vanilla extract
- ½ tsp cinnamon
- Pinch of salt
- ⅓ cup dairy-free chocolate chips

Directions:
1. In your food processor or blender, combine the chickpeas, nut butter, syrup, vanilla, cinnamon, and salt and process until smooth.
2. Transfer to a large bowl or food storage container and mix in the chocolate chips. Serve.

Nutrition: Calories: 363; Fat: 17g; Protein: 10g; Carbs: 43g

111. Green Smoothie Bowl with Berries
Preparation time: 5 minutes
Cooking time: 0 minutes
Servings: 2
Ingredients:

- 2 medium fresh or frozen bananas
- 2 cups chopped kale
- 1½ cups plain unsweetened almond milk
- 1½ cups fresh or frozen strawberries
- ½ avocado, peeled & pitted
- ½ cup rolled or instant oats
- 2 scoops whey protein powder
- ¼ cup sunflower seeds
- ¼ cup fresh berries of choice

Directions:
1. Combine the bananas, kale, almond milk, strawberries, avocado, oats, and whey in a blender. Process until smooth and pour into two bowls.
2. Top each bowl with the sunflower seeds and berries to serve.

Nutrition: Calories: 561; Fat: 20g; Protein: 36g; Carbs: 66g

112. Pineapple Breeze Smoothie
Preparation time: 5 minutes
Cooking time: 0 minutes
Servings: 1
Ingredients:

- 1 (1 oz) scoop of vanilla protein powder
- 1 tsp-size piece of fresh ginger
- 1 cup frozen spinach
- ½ cup store-bought chopped frozen pineapple chunks
- 1¼ cups unsweetened almond milk

Directions:
1. Place the protein powder, ginger, spinach, pineapple, and milk in the blender.
2. Process on high speed until smooth. Serve.

Nutrition: Calories: 148; Fat: 2g; Protein: 22g; Carbs: 12g

113. Blueberry-Banana Smoothie
Preparation time: 5 minutes
Cooking time: 0 minutes
Servings: 4
Ingredients:

- 3 cups sliced fresh or frozen bananas
- 3 cups fresh or frozen blueberries
- 2 cups spinach
- 2 scoops vanilla vegan protein powder
- 2 cups unsweetened vanilla almond milk
- 2 cups ice-cold water
- 1 cup orange juice

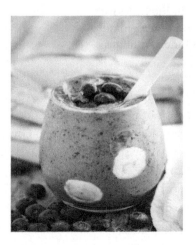

Directions:
1. Combine all the ingredients in your blender and process until

smooth. Serve.
Nutrition: Calories: 240; Fat: 4g; Protein: 11g; Carbs: 51g

114. Mint Chocolate Smoothie
Preparation time: 5 minutes
Cooking time: 0 minutes
Servings: 1
Ingredients:

- 1 (1-ounce) scoop of chocolate protein powder
- ¼ cup fresh mint leaves, loosely packed
- 1 cup frozen spinach
- 1 small frozen banana
- 1 tsp spirulina
- 1¼ cups unsweetened almond milk

Directions:
2. Place protein powder, mint, spinach, banana, spirulina, and milk in the blender.
3. Process on high speed until smooth. Serve.
Nutrition: Calories: 253; Fat: 5g; Protein: 24g; Carbs: 35g

115. Orange and Beet Protein Shake
Preparation time: 5 minutes
Cooking time: 0 minutes
Servings: 2
Ingredients:

- 2 cups water
- 2 cups beet greens
- 2 beets, peeled & diced
- 2 oranges, peeled
- 2 scoops vanilla protein powder
- Juice of ½ lemon

Directions:
1. Place the water, greens, beets, oranges, protein powder, and lemon juice into a blender.
2. Blend the ingredients until smooth. Serve.
Nutrition: Calories: 192; Fat: 0g; Protein: 25g; Carbs: 24g

116. Apple Pie Smoothie
Preparation time: 5 minutes
Cooking time: 0 minutes
Servings: 2
Ingredients:

- 2 large apples, cored
- 2 cups of reduced-fat milk
- 1 cup nonfat or low-fat plain Greek yogurt
- 1 cup baby spinach, packed
- 1 cup ice
- 2 scoops whey protein powder
- ¼ cup ground flaxseed
- 2 pitted dates

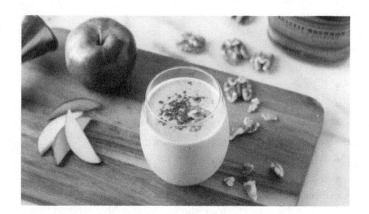

- 2 tsp avocado oil or extra-virgin olive oil
- ½ tsp ground cinnamon

Directions:
1. Add apples, milk, yogurt, spinach, ice, whey, flaxseed, dates, oil, and cinnamon in a blender.
2. Process on high until smooth. Serve.

Nutrition: Calories: 638; Fat: 17g; Protein: 52g; Carbs: 74g

117. Peanut Butter Banana Smoothie

Preparation time: 5 minutes
Cooking time: 0 minutes
Servings: 2
Ingredients:
- 1 medium banana
- 1½ cups skim milk
- ¾ cup nonfat or low-fat plain Greek yogurt
- 1 cup ice
- 2 scoops whey protein powder
- 2 tbsp peanut butter
- 2 tbsp ground flaxseed
- 1 tbsp maple syrup

Directions:
1. In a blender, combine the banana, milk, yogurt, ice, whey, peanut butter, flaxseed, and maple syrup.
2. Process on high until smooth. Serve.

Nutrition: Calories: 467; Fat: 13g; Protein: 48g; Carbs: 42g

118. Tropical Sunrise Smoothie

Preparation time: 5 minutes
Cooking time: 0 minutes
Servings: 4
Ingredients:
- 2 fresh or frozen bananas, chopped
- 2 cups frozen pineapple pieces
- 2 cups frozen mango pieces
- 2 scoops vanilla protein powder
- 4 tbsp hemp hearts
- 4 cups spinach
- 4 cups coconut water or filtered water

Directions:
1. Combine all the ingredients in your blender and process until smooth. Serve.

Nutrition: Calories: 227; Fat: 7g; Protein: 17g; Carbs: 36g

119. Pumpkin Spice Smoothie

Preparation time: 5 minutes
Cooking time: 0 minutes
Servings: 1
Ingredients:
- 1 (1 oz) scoop of vanilla protein powder
- ½ cup canned pumpkin purée
- 1 small frozen banana

- 1 tsp -size piece of fresh ginger
- 1 tsp -size piece of fresh turmeric
- ½ tsp cinnamon
- ¼ tsp nutmeg
- 2 tbsp hemp hearts
- 1 tsp ground flaxseed
- 1¼ cups unsweetened almond milk

Directions:
1. Place protein powder, pumpkin purée, banana, ginger, turmeric, cinnamon, nutmeg, hemp hearts, flaxseed, and milk in the blender.
2. Process on high speed until smooth, and serve.

Nutrition: Calories: 463; Fat: 19g; Protein: 31g; Carbs: 45g

120. Strawberry Cheesecake Smoothie

Preparation time: 5 minutes
Cooking time: 0 minutes
Servings: 2
Ingredients:

- 2 cups frozen strawberries
- 2½ cups reduced-fat milk
- 1½ cups nonfat or low-fat plain Greek yogurt
- 2 scoops whey protein powder
- 4 tbsp low-fat cream cheese

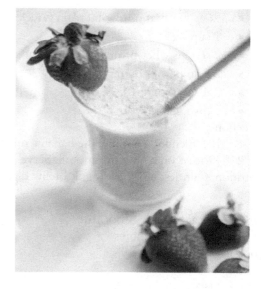

Directions:
1. In a blender, combine the strawberries, milk, yogurt, whey, and cream cheese.
2. Process on high until smooth. Serve.

Nutrition: Calories: 537; Fat: 13g; Protein: 58g; Carbs: 48g

30-DAY MEAL PLAN

DAY	BREAKFAST	LUNCH	DINNER	SNACKS/ DESSERTS
1	Banana Chia Overnight Oats	Grilled Greek Chicken Kabobs	Pork Chops with Mushroom Sauce	Sweet Potato Nachos
2	Classic Tofu Scramble	Steak-Spiced Tofu with Asparagus	Cod Fillet with Charred Tomatillo Salsa	Blueberry Cheesecake Cup
3	Blueberry Cobbler Oatmeal	Ginger Beef Sirloin and Bok Choy	Mustard Almond-Crusted Chicken Breast	Vanilla Hemp Protein Bars
4	Tempeh & Kale Breakfast Skillet	Cauliflower Fried Rice	Pork Meatball, Greens, and Beans Skillet	Chickpea Choco Cookie Dough
5	Eggs and Tomato Breakfast Melts	Feta Turkey Burgers	Shrimp Scampi with Whole-Grain Pasta	Turmeric Popcorn
6	Breakfast Greek Yogurt Parfait	Lemon-Garlic Cod with Asparagus	Beef and Bean Chili	Bacon-Flavored Coconut Chips
7	Sausage-Egg Scramble	Quinoa & Chickpea Tabbouleh	Deconstructed Turkey Lasagna	Vanilla Almond Truffles
8	Apple-Oat Protein Muffins	Ginger-Hoisin Pork Wraps	Lentil and Zucchini Pasta Bake	Stuffed Avocado
9	Breakfast Spinach Shakshuka	Loaded Sweet Potatoes	Blackened Baked Tilapia Fillet	Blueberry PB Muffins
10	Egg and Canadian Bacon Cups	Three-Bean Salad	Spiced Pork Medallions with Apples	High-Protein Crab Balls
11	Baked Eggs with Smoked Salmon	Zucchini Pizza Boats	Baked Tamari Salmon and Zucchini	Lemon Drop Energy Balls
12	Vanilla Protein Crepes	Green Chicken Enchiladas	Black Bean Burgers	Pb & Banana Collard Green Wraps
13	Ham and Feta Quiche	Tuna Power Wrap	Flank Steak with Brussels Sprouts	Poached Caramel Peaches
14	Egg, And Spinach Burrito	Pork Souvlaki with Yogurt-Dill Dip	Deconstructed Cabbage Roll Stew	Smoky Tofu Bites

15	Banana-Nut Pancakes	Crispy Tofu and Chickpea Bowl	Dijon Mustard Baked Scallops	Pineapple Spice Sorbet
16	Spinach-Tomato Frittata	Vegetable and Beef Skewers	Black Bean Quinoa Casserole	Cinnamon-Roasted Chickpeas
17	Vanilla Blueberry Overnight Oats	Salmon Salad Wrap	Lamb Shepherd's Pie	Very Berry Ice Cream
18	Sweet Potato and Turkey Hash	Veggie Fried Rice	Tofu & Veggie Tray Bake	Coconut-Cranberry Trail Mix
19	Cottage Cheese Berry Bowl	Lettuce Wraps with Smoked Tofu	Adobo Sirloin Steak	Chocolate Peanut Butter Cups
20	Protein-Packed French Toast	Baked Panko-Breaded Pork Chops	Garlic Salmon, Sweet Potato, and Broccoli	Tofu Chili Fries
21	Banana Chia Overnight Oats	Grilled Greek Chicken Kabobs	Pork Chops with Mushroom Sauce	Chocolate Banana Nice Cream
22	Classic Tofu Scramble	Steak-Spiced Tofu with Asparagus	Cod Fillet with Charred Tomatillo Salsa	Endive Hummus & Hemp Boats
23	Blueberry Cobbler Oatmeal	Ginger Beef Sirloin and Bok Choy	Mustard Almond-Crusted Chicken Breast	Broiled Grapefruit with Yogurt
24	Tempeh & Kale Breakfast Skillet	Cauliflower Fried Rice	Pork Meatball, Greens, and Beans Skillet	Tofu Nori Wraps
25	Eggs and Tomato Breakfast Melts	Feta Turkey Burgers	Shrimp Scampi with Whole-Grain Pasta	Protein-Packed Rice Pudding
26	Breakfast Greek Yogurt Parfait	Lemon-Garlic Cod with Asparagus	Beef and Bean Chili	Apple Cinnamon Stacks
27	Sausage-Egg Scramble	Quinoa & Chickpea Tabbouleh	Deconstructed Turkey Lasagna	Black Bean Brownie Mug Cake
28	Apple-Oat Protein Muffins	Ginger-Hoisin Pork Wraps	Lentil and Zucchini Pasta Bake	Tuna Salad Rice Cakes
29	Breakfast Spinach Shakshuka	Loaded Sweet Potatoes	Blackened Baked Tilapia Fillet	Almond Butter Protein Bites
30	Egg and Canadian Bacon Cups	Three-Bean Salad	Spiced Pork Medallions with Apples	Cocoa-Cranberry Energy Balls

Volume Equivalents (Liquid)

US STANDARD	US STANDARD (OUNCES)	METRIC (APPROXIMATE)
2 tablespoons	1 fl. oz.	30 mL
¼ cup	2 fl. oz.	60 mL
½ cup	4 fl. oz.	120 mL
1 cup	8 fl. oz.	240 mL
1½ cups	12 fl. oz.	355 mL
2 cups or 1 pint	16 fl. oz.	475 mL
4 cups or 1 quart	32 fl. oz.	1 L
1 gallon	128 fl. oz.	4 L

Volume Equivalents (Dry)

US STANDARD	METRIC (APPROXIMATE)
⅛ teaspoon	0.5 mL
¼ teaspoon	1 mL
½ teaspoon	2 mL
¾ teaspoon	4 mL
1 teaspoon	5 mL
1 tablespoon	15 mL
¼ cup	59 mL
⅓ cup	79 mL
½ cup	118 mL
⅔ cup	156 mL
¾ cup	177 mL
1 cup	235 mL
2 cups or 1 pint	475 mL
3 cups	700 mL
4 cups or 1 quart	1 L
½ gallon	2 L
1 gallon	4 L

Oven Temperatures

FAHRENHEIT (F)	CELSIUS (C) (APPROXIMATE)
250	120
300	150
325	165
350	180
375	190
400	200
425	220
450	230

Weight Equivalents

US STANDARD	METRIC (APPROXIMATE)
½ ounce	15 g
1 ounce	30 g
2 ounces	60 g
4 ounces	115 g
8 ounces	225 g
12 ounces	340 g
16 ounces or 1 pound	455 g

Conclusion

Women have different dietary needs than men when it comes to bodybuilding. And to get the most out of your routine and diet, you need something specific to you. That's why a cookbook tailored especially towards women, which contains both easy and healthy recipes, can make all the difference. Bodybuilding Cookbook for Women is designed for readers who want to look and feel better. The comprehensive information in this book will provide readers with everything they need to build a healthier body and transform their lifestyle. It contains over 120 tasty, easy-to-prepare recipes along with detailed instructions and nutritional information. There is also a 30-day meal plan provided to help readers become the strongest, healthiest version of themselves.

More importantly, it offers a comprehensive resource to help women achieve their physical goals while simultaneously nourishing their bodies and spirit. With tips, tricks, and advice to maximize results and minimize efforts, this cookbook will help you gain the strength and confidence to achieve the body of your dreams and the lifestyle you've always wanted.

Looking back on the things we've discussed in this cookbook, for women, the bodybuilding diet plan can have some slight modifications from the traditional diet plan as a result of a number of reasons. Our bodies can absorb and utilize certain vitamins, minerals, and nutrients differently than men. To get the most out of your bodybuilding goals, it's important to monitor the foods that you eat and ensure that you're getting all the necessary nutrients. Women should focus on macro and micronutrients and use supplements to support their bodybuilding goals. It is also important to remember that proper hydration and rest in addition to proper nutrition, are key to successful bodybuilding.

Women also need more calcium and vitamin D, which can be obtained from a healthy diet of fruits, vegetables, nuts, and seeds. This helps to maintain good bone health and general well-being. For optimal energy, consuming nutrient-dense meals, avoiding processed food, and dietary restrictions should be taken into account. It is also important to develop a healthy lifestyle, both in terms of physical energy and emotional well-being. Regular exercise coupled with a nutritious diet can help ensure optimal health and well-being.

We've also discussed the three macronutrients carbohydrates, proteins, and fats—and their essential roles in bodybuilding. To maintain a healthy and balanced diet according to your bodybuilding goals, it's important to ensure your diet provides adequate sources of the three macronutrients in the correct proportions. The primary sources of carbohydrates are grains, cereals, fruits, and vegetables. To meet your protein needs, ensure that you consume animal proteins such as eggs, milk, and lean meats. Fats can be obtained from plant-based foods like nuts, seeds, and avocados, as well as from healthy oils such as olive and coconut oil. Finally, don't forget to monitor your daily caloric intake and try to limit your intake of refined sugars and processed foods. Another important thing to consider is the bulking and cutting cycles for fat loss and muscle growth. Bulking and cutting cycles involve following a meal plan for a certain amount of time that combines higher caloric intake and more intense exercises when bulking and lower caloric intake with more endurance exercises when cutting. Bulking and cutting cycles are designed to help you reach your desired body composition in the quickest and safest manner possible.

The maintenance phase of bodybuilding is when you focus on maintaining your healthy physique and weight. During this phase, you should be mindful of your macros and adjust your diet according to your changing body composition. This phase is an important part of the bodybuilding journey and can help you maintain a healthy lifestyle and body composition. Furthermore, it is important to take breaks from your workouts from time to time to prevent burnout and help with recovery.

So, why make a healthy switch? Not only does a healthy diet and lifestyle help with bodybuilding goals, but it also helps improve one's overall health and well-being. Good nutrition helps to fuel up for workouts, promoting an active and healthy lifestyle. Furthermore, a balanced diet helps to ward off diseases by providing the body with all the essential nutrients it needs to stay healthy. Finally, focusing on nutrition also promotes better mental health as it can help reduce stress levels and improve mood. Not only is a healthy body necessary to get the most out of your bodybuilding journey and workouts, but it also helps to keep you energized and focused. With the right food, supplements, and sleep, you can attain your desired body and strength in a relatively short amount of time.

Some of the tips we've also given are to use a macro-counting app to track your meals and make sure you're consuming just the right number of macronutrients to reach your bodybuilding goals. You can try using MyFitnessPal or MyMacros+ to help you stay on track. Proper hydration is also important for bodybuilding. Not only does it help provide essential electrolytes for muscle growth, but it also helps reduce fatigue and muscle cramps from intense workouts. Meal prepping can be a huge time-saver, and make sure that you're not struggling to cook or eat on a regular basis. Additionally, meal prepping can help you stay on track with your macros, ensuring that you're getting all the nutrients your body needs to build muscle.

Additionally, listening to your body also encourages proper rest and recovery. As a bodybuilder, it is important to listen to your body so that you can adjust your diet and workouts depending on how you are feeling. It is important to give your body time to rest and recover as it is the key to building muscle. Allowing your body time to recover can help reduce fatigue, improve strength, and help improve overall performance. Lastly, consult with a doctor or nutritionist before starting any new diet or bodybuilding program, as they can help you determine the best course of action for your individual health and body. It is always a good idea to speak to someone about your goals and what you are looking to accomplish before starting a new diet or workout plan. Remember, there is no one-size-fits-all when it comes to nutrition and bodybuilding, so be sure to consult with a professional before making any major changes.

And now, we hope this book can help guide you towards a better lifestyle that involves healthy eating habits, an active routine, proper rest and recovery, and the appropriate supplements. The combination of all these factors can help you maintain better health and reach your bodybuilding goals in the most efficient way possible. A well-rounded diet, exercise program, and recovery plan can help you create a lasting transformation and foster a healthier, happier life. Therefore, take the time to build up your body, eat well and make a positive change to improve your overall well-being.

Made in the USA
Las Vegas, NV
29 December 2023

83675489R00046